PSYCHOLOGY LIBRARY EDITIONS:
CHILD DEVELOPMENT

Volume 4

PSYCHOLOGICAL DEVELOPMENT OF HIGH RISK MULTIPLE BIRTH CHILDREN

PSYCHOLOGICAL DEVELOPMENT OF HIGH RISK MULTIPLE BIRTH CHILDREN

VITA KRALL AND SHERMAN C. FEINSTEIN

Routledge
Taylor & Francis Group
LONDON AND NEW YORK

First published in 1991 by Harwood Academic Publishers

This edition first published in 2018
by Routledge
2 Park Square, Milton Park, Abingdon, Oxon OX14 4RN

and by Routledge
711 Third Avenue, New York, NY 10017

Routledge is an imprint of the Taylor & Francis Group, an informa business

British Library Cataloguing in Publication Data
A catalogue record for this book is available from the British Library

ISBN: 978-1-138-74142-3 (Set)
ISBN: 978-1-351-27384-8 (Set) (ebk)
ISBN: 978-1-138-09348-5 (Volume 4) (hbk)
ISBN: 978-1-315-10679-3 (Volume 4) (ebk)

Publisher's Note
The publisher has gone to great lengths to ensure the quality of this reprint but points out that some imperfections in the original copies may be apparent.

Disclaimer
The publisher has made every effort to trace copyright holders and would welcome correspondence from those they have been unable to trace.

PSYCHOLOGICAL DEVELOPMENT OF HIGH RISK MULTIPLE BIRTH CHILDREN

Vita Krall, PhD
Milford, Connecticut

and

Sherman C. Feinstein, MD
Michael Reese Hospital and Medical Center
Chicago, Illinois

harwood academic publishers
chur • london • paris • new york • melbourne

Harwood Academic Publishers

Post Office Box 197
London WC2E 9PX
United Kingdom

58, rue Lhomond
75005 Paris
France

Post Office Box 786
Cooper Station
New York, New York 10276
United States of America

Private Bag 8
Camberwell, Victoria 3124
Australia

Library of Congress Cataloging-in-Publication Data

Krall, Vita.
Psychological development of high risk multiple birth children / by Vita Krall and Sherman C. Feinstein.
p. cm.
ISBN 3-7186-0516-3 (hardcover)
1. Child development—Longitudinal studies. 2. Birth, Multiple—Longitudinal studies. I. Feinstein, Sherman C. II. Title.
[DNLM: 1. Longitudinal Studies—United States. 2. Pregnancy, Multiple. 3. Quadruplets. 4. Quintuplets. 5. Triplets. WQ 235 K89p]
RJ131.K72 1991
155.44′4—dc20
DNLM/DLC 90-4688

To the parents and children

Contents

Preface

This book is a report of a longitudinal study of multiple birth children including quintuplets, quadruplets and triplets. The children in this study are the product of fertility drugs and come from five different upper socio-economic families.

We were interested in the development of these children since, for at least two of the families, the infants were quite premature and/or smaller than average. In addition, because of the need for multiple caretaking in the early months of life, we had additional theoretical interests in their bonding and attachment. The theoretical questions that arose included whether development would be delayed because of their prematurity and possible problems with attachment. The literature available on prematurity suggests that there are later effects on development in low birthweight children. Previous studies on other multiples, such as twins, concerned themselves with separation-individuation and the development of separate identities in multiple birth children. This book, however, addresses the emotional and personality states of these children in relation to their multiple birth status.

The children were tested every three months until age two, and then at six month intervals until age three. They were tested again on a yearly basis through age nine, with one family follow-up at age twelve. Until age two they were administered the Bayley infant scales and the Décarie object-constancy and object-relations tests. Between age two and age five they were administered the Stanford-Binet, Form L-M intelligence test, and human figure drawings. From age six through age twelve these tests included the Wechsler Intelligence Scale for Children, Revised; the Rorschach ink blot test; and additional human figure drawings.

The test results indicated that an infant's development became normative by age two, with the higher birthweight children catching up slightly earlier. Mental scales increased above the level of the motor scores on the Bayley. Objectal development, or attachment, as measured by the Décarie, preceded object constancy in the early infancy of these multiple birth children. It suggested that multiple caretaking in these early months did not interfere with the attachment to the mother. There was a high correlation between objectal development and intellectual development. Some motor development problems and later academic difficulties were found in cohorts regardless of initial birthweight. Emotionally, these children were found to show greater control and less impulsivity as a group than a standardization sample. The children also showed good individuation and adequacy of emotional development.

Acknowledgements

We should like to acknowledge the generous and gracious support and involvement of the families who participated in this study, without whom this project would not have been possible.

We should also like to acknowledge the generous support of the Arlene and Marshall Bennett Laboratory for Child Psychiatry Research of the Michael Reese Hospital and Medical Center.

Thanks also to the tireless dedication and work of the following examiners who participated in the collection of the test data: Dennis Kennedy, PhD; Jerrie Ann Will, PhD; Barbara Rayson, MA; and Floyd S. Irvin, PhD.

CHAPTER 1

Introduction and Review of the Literature

Multiple births remain one of nature's most fascinating and revealing phenomena. Usually considered a delightful, curious event, the birth of twins and other multiples (Scheinfeld, 1967) actually activates numerous biological, sociocultural, and psychological dimensions. This report describes the results of a longitudinal investigation of multiple birth children; quintuplets, quadruplets, and triplets studied over twelve years by a team of behavioral scientists from the Arlene and Marshall Bennett Laboratory for Child Psychiatry Research, Michael Reese Hospital and Medical Center and The Pritzker School of Medicine, University of Chicago. The project began with the opportunity to study a set of quintuplets born to a couple who had been treated with human menopausal gonadotropins as part of a fertility study. Subsequent families were added to the longitudinal study project after fulfillment of the research criteria concerning age and availability.

Prior to the use of the hormone drugs to induce pregnancy, the occurrence of multiple births beyond twins was rare. There is a large literature on twins as multiples, but little data on multiples beyond twins (Scheinfeld, 1967; review of Psychological Abstracts, 1972–1988). A major scientific emphasis in the study of twins has been comparison of monozygotic and dizygotic twins for the purpose of determining concordance or discordance for various traits or psychopathology (schizophrenia) (Feinstein, 1985). These studies have made important contributions to the understanding of genetic influence, particularly in the area of psychopathology. It was apparent to us, however, that our particular cohort would not lend itself to this type of scientific research. Our children were born as a result of fertility drugs and, hence, are all fraternal (born from multiple eggs). It would also not be possible to assume that their environments would be equal, since multiple parenting would certainly be necessary from very early infancy.

Multiple birth infants are often premature and of low birth weight (Feinstein, 1985), as were our earliest subjects. It seemed important to design a protocol that would trace these infants' early development. There was considerable interest in the pediatric literature then and now as to the outcome of such infants and the ability to predict outcome for premature and low birth weight infants. We asked the question: How do low birth weight and premature infants fare, given the best care by parents who wanted them and had the ability to provide. Studies on low birth weight and premature infants (Sigman, & Parmalee, 1979) often included a large number of cases from lower socioeconomic families whose care had not been optimal.

We also were interested in the nature of the attachment of such low birthweight and premature infants to their mothers given their multiple birth status and the probability that there would be multiple parenting. Did multiple caretaking, particularly in the first year of life, interfere with the development of specific bonding to the mother and later development of object relationships? Did the multiple birth and multiple caretaking situation interfere with later personality development, particularly the development of a cohesive sense of self?

Our basic cohort of subjects are all fraternal and, hence, do not provide the opportunity to compare genetic and environmental influence. The probability is that in each group the amount of similarity between the multiples is no more than that between siblings of different age. However, the literature on twin comparisons can be of considerable help in evaluating the information obtained on our fraternal multiples.

MENTAL DEVELOPMENT

The publications of the Louisville Twin Study offer important information on the risk factors of prematurity and low birth weight as these affect mental development (Wilson, 1985). Their data "showed no evidence of a long-term deficit in mental development assignable to low birth weight by itself." When low birth weight twins were matched with their higher birth weight twin, "there was no significant deficit in mental functioning." "If there was a residual effect, it was subtle indeed and was not detected by a standard intelligence test". They did find, however, that a combination of both very low birth weight and early delivery did seem to be related to some long-term deficit in IQ; but a large proportion of these infants were found to have come from low SES homes. They examined two possible explanations for any effect that low birth weight might have on mental functioning: poor prenatal nutrition or a symptom of a broader constellation of deficiencies. Nutrition is related to other variables such as socioeconomic status and postnatal care. The other hypothesis attempts to explain decrements on the basis of a genetic link to the prematurity status itself: that is, infants are being born who in previous times might have aborted because of other related deficiencies.

These findings support a genetic hypothesis for mental development, even when prematurity and/or low birth weight are involved. Other work (Wilson & Matheny, 1983) finds a very strong link between mental development and parental intellectual level, as measured by educational level of the mother. They do not deny the importance of an effective learning environment.

On the basis of these findings, we might have predicted (had these data been available in 1973 when our study was begun), that our low birthweight and premature infants would eventually catch up and become normative. Our initial findings, reported in 1980 (Krall, Feinstein, & Kennedy, 1980) that both scores adjusted for gestation and unadjusted scores were highly correlated with birth weight in the initial months. There was "catch up" by two years, after an initial lag in development. The question has persisted in the singleton literature for premature and low birthweight infants as to whether there are subtle residuals that will demonstrate themselves in later school years in other than IQ level.

Our infants came from upper socioeconomic families, where mother's educational level was on the average college or above college level. We can assume both good nutritional care, as well as emotional care as based on the parental desire to have these children. A related question about intellectual development might be whether there was an equal environment in terms of stimulation for children within cohorts. Ainslie, Olmstead, and O'Loughlin (1987) question the equal environmental hypothesis for twins and suggest that parents tend to respond to slight differences in their twins, maximizing them as it were to aid in telling them apart.

ATTACHMENT

A number of studies related to the behavior of newborn twins, both full term and premature, and their attachment to the mother (Riese,

1983, 1984, 1988; Goldberg, Perrotta, Minde & Corter, 1986), and sex differences in the attachment of twins (Brooks & Lewis, 1974). Riese found a similarity in behavior within twin pairs suggesting a constitutional or genetic influence on certain behavior patterns during the neonatal period (irritability, resistance to soothing, reactivity, and reinforcement value). There was a decrease in individual consistency of scores as prematurity increased. Riese suggests that this might mean that the parent would be given "mixed signals" for parenting. In addition, full term infants were more resistant to soothing, and there were also differences in degrees of reactivity, irritability, and activity level during active sleep. Singleton full-term infants were reported by Kurzberg and associates (Kurzberg, Vaugham, Jr., Daum, Grellong, Albin, & Rotkin, 1979) to have higher performance on the visual following and auditory orienting items than low-birthweight infants.

These findings suggest that the preterm infant presents a lower level of arousal in these areas of behavior: activity level, visual following, auditory orienting, and irritability, and a quicker response to soothing. In one sense, this makes the task for the caregiver easier. In another sense, the infant does not stimulate caregiving behavior from the caretaker as well. Also, it has been found that alert and responsive infants have been shown to have more responsive and stimulating mothers (Osofsky, 1976). When there is more than one infant to be cared for as in the multiple situation, the less alert and active infant is less likely to be attended to by the caretaker.

The nature of attachment in full term and preterm twins has been addressed by Goldberg and associates (1986). In their study, a majority of low-birth-weight twins and singletons were securely attached as measured by the strange situation (Ainsworth, Blehar, Waters, & Wall, 1978). Ainsworth et al. (1978) found that mothers in securely attached full term dyads were rated in the first year as being more sensitive, accepting, accessible, and cooperative than those of the less securely attached infants. Goldberg et al. found some inconsistency in their findings for preterm infants. Ratings of maternal behavior were related to subsequent attachment, but ratings of infant behavior were not. It was suggested that the maternal ratings captured the appropriateness of maternal response and the dyadic relationship, and that the infant behaviors would not be expected to do so. Mothers who were found to be securely attached to their preterm infants were rated as more attentive and responsive to their infants at all ages, on all scales (sensitivity, acceptance, accessibility, and cooperation).

Szajnberg, Skrinjaric, and Moore (1989), studying attunement and attachment in monozygotic and dizygotic twins at eleven months of age, found no significant relationship between attunement and attachment. However, he pointed out that this is an evolving phenomenon. An infant who is a high affect signaler with a low responding mother, may become a low affect signaler if mother persists: "if there is sufficient interaction between mother and infant, attunement rate may vary with time".

There was some differential patterning found for Goldberg's preterm infants as compared with the Ainsworth et al. full-term sample. Goldberg et al. found a reversal for the marginal and insecure attachment groups. One possibility might have been that the marginal group was misplaced with the secure group in the normative sample. Another possibility was that finding the predicted pattern from secure to marginal to insecure only at six weeks might indicate the importance of the early weeks of life in shaping attachment. Another possible explanation for the difference they found in patterning for the preterms might be that for the preterm the mother might be rated low in sensitivity for giving a great deal of auditory stimulation, for example. In other words, qualitatively different forms of maternal relatedness might be necessary to arouse the preterm infant. Another possible explanation given that is quite pertinent to our own subjects, is that for the twins in their preterm group, peer attachment and the presence of a secondary caretaker might have made up some for the diminished capacity of the maternal caretaker. They suggest that without these additional attachments they might have been in the insecurely attached group.

Since our subjects were all fraternal, sex differences in attachment would be of interest. Brooks and Lewis (1974) studied thirteen-month-old, opposite-sex twins. They found that girl twins touch, look at, and seek proximity with their mothers significantly more than do their brothers. These results seem to be related to the sex-appropriate teaching of the mothers. They suggest that maternal socialization minimizes the proximal behaviors exhibited by mother and son, while not restricting mother-daughter interaction. Brief separations from the mother were then found to affect the boys' but not the girls' subsequent attachment behaviors. The boys seen second exhibited significantly more proximal behaviors. They state that these same sex differences have been reported for singletons.

Specific influences that the multiple birth has on the parental relationship with the infants have been discussed by Showers & McCleery

(1984). Because twins and other multiples may be separated after birth, with one or more infants remaining in the hospital for a time, there may be some interference with bonding with those infants. Hay and O'Brien (1987) found that depression and maladaptive behavior to classroom peers were much more common among those twins discharged from hospital after the cotwin. The parent may attach to the infant taken home, or later become more caring of the weaker infant on return. Szajnberg et al. (1989) found that mothers reported compensating by not attuning to their favored twin. Subsequent influences can be preferences for one or another child and attribution of positive and negative features to different children. Eventually the child may respond by attaching to other caretakers, such as grandparents, which can have a positive effect by facilitating differentiation.

PSYCHIATRIC OUTCOME

A frequent patterning that is reported for twins is a dominance-submissiveness relationship. One retrospective study of twins (Paluszny & Abelson, 1975) has shown that a large number of twins seen in a psychiatric clinic came in for dependency problems. However, there were only half as many twins referred to clinic than would be expected from their occurrence in the general population. One explanation for this finding might be the submissive-dependent relationship is not always a permanent one in any individual twinship and does not always present a problem requiring psychiatric referral. Twins are also described as having role-switching relationships, in which in one type of activity one twin is dominant and in another type of activity the other twin is dominant (Anderson, 1985). Anderson points out that the unique advantage of having a twin is often not emphasized enough. In role switching, each twin (or in the case of larger multiples, siblings) may take turns acting as a model in behaviors in which they excel. The potentiality for empathy and the understanding of a peer of the same developmental age may also be important environmentally for stimulating personal growth. The very need to compete and interact with each other may stimulate the capacity for social interrelationships.

However, in large sample studies of dominance and submissiveness in twins, Moilanen (1987, 1988) reports that submissive twins tended to have more psychosomatic symptoms, and dominant twins tended to have more nervous complaints. They explain the somatic complaints on the basis of having to adapt and be obedient, and the depression on the basis of few opportunities to feel successful, i.e. feelings of inferiority. The nervous complaints are explained by the need always to be active.

LANGUAGE DEVELOPMENT

Some research studies maintain that multiples tend to lag behind singletons in articulation and syntax elements of speech, and language development. Hay, Prior, Collett, and Williams (1987) report that at the age of 30 months, twin boys were 8 months behind matched singletons and twin girls on expressive language, and 6 months behind on verbal comprehension. They were also 5 months behind on symbolic play and this delay was closely related to language. The twin boys also had more articulation problems. Conway, Lytton, and Pysh (1980) report that three-year-old twins speak less than singletons of similar age. They formulate sentence component phrases as competently as singletons, but these tend to be shorter and less frequently expressed in sentences. Mothers of twins are reported to speak to the twins less, and in shorter, and less complex utterances than mothers of singletons. Therefore, there is less verbal interaction between child and mother. Biological handicap accounted for less influence on these findings than did the reduced opportunity for communication with adults. The reduction of opportunities were attributed both to the fact that the child shares parental attention with its twin and the reduced environmental facilitation of using phrases in sentence formation.

Tomasello, Mannle, & Kruger (1986) studied younger twins and singletons of fifteen months when crucial language environments are being developed. They were interested in whether the need for twins to share the language environment, that is the triadic situation, contributed to the delay in twin speech. They were also interested in whether the caretaking at this particular age, the need for more directive relationship between mother and child, would influence the type of speech engaged in by the child, that is a more expressive rather than a referential style of speech. Expressive speech is, they assert, marked by slower linguistic development. They found that the twins of their study engaged in very little dyadic, joint interaction with their mothers and were less often directly addressed by mother. They attribute these differences to the nature of the triadic relationship between mother and twins, the mother having to share her utterances with two children. They also found that mothers of twins had a more directive style of language with their children. They attribute this finding to the pressure of the mother of twins having to take care of two children of about one year of age rather than one. The result of this directiveness is an increase of expressive speech. Also the mothers of twins engaged in less topic continuances than imitations, which would be related to slower and less productivity of language on the part of the child. This, also, they believe, is related again to the triadic situation. Mother needs to pay attention to both and to manage a more complex child behavioral situation.

ACADEMIC OUTCOME

The Australian twin study, (Johnston, Prior, & Hay, 1984), has reported reading delay, particularly in decoding, among twin males of high intelligence as measured by the performance scale of the WISC-R. They report data that relates this delay to preschool language problems. Reading comprehension appears to be better in this group, which they attribute to an ability to compensate on the basis of their advanced performance scores.

The Louisville Twin Study (Matheny, Dolan, & Wilson, 1976), measured antecedent factors to academic difficulties in a large group of twins. The children were selected to have academic difficulties by teachers or guidance counselors. The index twins compared with a matched control sample were found to be overly active, distractible, temperamental, and having sleep and feeding problems. The concordance rates for identical as compared with fraternal twins suggested a biological component to some of these findings. These rates were greater for sleeping and feeding problems and activity level, and lower for speech articulation errors, distractibility, and temperament. The achievement test measures differentiated the index twins from the control twins better than did the ability measures. The authors suggest that the behavioral syndrome of activity and temperament, and disturbances in bodily function interfered with children of average ability to learn and retain academic subjects.

The question of whether there are biological bases to these academic findings has been further raised. The concordance rates suggest genetic factors. The greater incidence of males having difficulties suggest a sex conditioning etiology. The authors also report a higher incidence of breech presentation and a lower rate of weight gain. Dolan and Matheny (1978) have gone on to study the rate of weight gain in these children. They have found a relatively slower rate of gain in weight for children with academic difficulties during the first two years of life. Chronic or acute disease did not seem to account for this downward trend. The authors speculate whether it is genetic influence on the timing of physical development or whether these findings can be related to the feeding problems noted in the previous study. The feeding problems themselves, however, might be explained as indirect expressions of faulty biological processes in the first two years, or that these children might be generally "immature." A complex etiology of genetic and both prenatal and postnatal factors may be involved in all of these findings. For example, as noted, the delayed language development has been found to be related to the social language environment of twins.

PERSONALITY DEVELOPMENT

It has been of interest whether the early prenatal and postnatal conditions of multiples not only affect cognitive, language, and academic functioning in later life, but also general personality style. Cohen, Allen, Pollin, Inoff, Werner, & Dibble (1972) have studied twins longitudinally with many personality, behavioral, and family measures. They find that the better endowed newborn developed into the more secure, trusting, and developmentally advanced child during the first year of life and an assertive, actively coping and competent toddler. The less well endowed children are described as more fearful of strangers and dependent on their mothers. Style of play was less well organized and included more gross play, frenetic activity, and relatively immature tactile activities. The authors emphasize the special importance of early differences in arousal and attention patterns in shaping early development. They also emphasize the importance of family responses to these constitutional aspects of the newborn. The more easily consoled and attentive child may be more easily engaged by the parent. While the weaker infant may gain more attention at times and be closer to mother for this reason, they may also be less competent in social skills with poorer language development.

Ainslee (1985) has emphasized the importance of early postnatal experiences and the first year of life, with the subphases of separation-individuation as being crucial in personality development. Early infancy problems necessitating separation from mother may influence early bonding conditions and may interfere with the natural synchrony of the early relationship and its reciprocity. Need to care simultaneously for two infants may stress and fatigue the mother, and present frustrating conditions, for example, in feeding for both mother and child. The symbiotic phase may be complicated by the fact that the relationship is not only with the mother but with the twin, which may interfere with the maternal bond. The other twin may become a source of attachment, a "transitional object" used for soothing. Some special problems of twins are variously referred to as "twinning," "mutual interidentification," or the "we-self." Problems of dependency and thinking of the self as part of a unit, and complementarity are further twin problems that are reported. Ainslee suggests that factors that assist twins in their separation and individuation are differential parental attachments and competition. Competition, he found, led to differentiation, and differentiation circularly led to competition. Ainslee emphasizes that the nature of zygosity of the twinship is less important in the way the infant negotiates the separation-individuation phases than the psychological circumstances of the particular twinship and family environment.

Some of these variations may relate to the extent to which the family treats the children as a unit and differentiates them (Goshen-Gottstein, 1980). Lower socioeconomic status may interfere with the capacity of parents to treat their twins differentially (Terry, 1975). Parents may form differential relationships with the twins based on a prenatal name chosen, postnatal similarities and differences, or physical likenesses to other family members. Parents may also differentiate the children based on the strength or weaknesses of the individual infants. This can then move the infants into complementary roles of "strong" and "weak," dominant or submissive. The children's own abilities may have an influence on the development of role relationships where one child maintains dominance in one activity and the other in other activities. We have mentioned role switching and the effect of competition on differentiation.

The extent of interidentification and lack of differentiation from the twin unit may create separation problems and later adult problems with intimacy and social relationships (Siemon, 1980). There can be separation anxiety, anger, and grief as the twin attempts to separate and to move into other relationships. Ainslee (1985) emphasizes, however, that one needs to differentiate between closeness and interdependence. Some of his twins maintained close ties, but had also attained psychological independence. He found adolescence an important time of differentiation for his sample of twins since they had to separate from parental figures and from each other. He found that many twins gave up the twinship as a primary relationship at that time. Other reconsolidated it, although on different terms. And for some it was a gradual process of differentiation over years.

The self-psychology theoretical literature may be helpful in understanding this developmental process. Von Broembsen (1988) has described the personality development of twinships. He states that the twin is half-way between a self-object and a transitional object. He describes two axes: the merger-separation-integration axis, and the activity-passivity axis in the separation-individuation process of the twinship. He emphasizes the importance of each twin being in synchrony in their developmental phase with regard to both axes. Von Broembsen (1988) lists four points on the separation-individuation continuum:

1. Merger strivings intersect with activity trends: nurturant, affiliative attitude.
2. Merger strivings intersect with passive trends: succorant attitude.
3. Separation strivings intersect with passive trends: passive-aggressive, entitled attitude.
4. Separation strivings intersect with active trends: constructive, assertive attitude.

The importance of the active-passive axis and the phallic aggressive personality component in analysis of adult male twins is emphasized by Ablon, Harrison, Valenstein, and Gifford (1986).

The intertwin identification process has been studied by comparing identical and fraternal twins with personality tests: a drawing task, and the Rorschach ink blot test. Rehmann (1979) had pairs of identical and fraternal twins do conjoint drawings. Identical twins, she found, show more anxiety and exhibit more rivalry. The fraternal twins were able to move graphically in and out of each other's space, complemented each other's imagery, and were able to draw separately.

Basit (1972) and Hamilton, Blewett, and Sydaha (1971) found marked similarities in the records of identical twins as compared with fraternal twins on the Rorschach ink blot test. In the Basit study, the significant differences were in M, FM, F%, FC and A.R.T. The Hamilton et al. study found differences in M, D, W%, R, Sum C, F%, and verbal output as measured by word count relative to R. The consistency in these findings on basic determinants suggests greater intertwin similarity in identical twins, and greater variation in fraternal twins in personality determinants. This further suggests greater ability on the part of fraternal twins to differentiate themselves.

HYPOTHESES

The following hypotheses might be made for our multiple birth children:

(1) We expected to find a differential between our low birth weight cohorts and our higher birth weight cohorts on the developmental mental and motor scales. Our pilot study (Krall, Feinstein, & Kennedy, 1980) suggested "catch up" by approximately two years of age.
(2) We did not expect to find interference with the maternal attachment in our multiples, regardless of the amount of multiple caretaking, because of the extent to which the mothers themselves were involved and concerned with that care. Schaffer (1963) suggested the capacity for many nonspecific attachments prior to maternal bonding in infants.
(3) We expected to find some language delay relative to norms for singletons.
(4) The above reports suggest that there may be residuals in the high risk infant that are expressed in learning difficulties, which may be masked by using adjusted developmental measures during the first three years.
(5) Personality measures should show differentiation and individual development in our multiples, since they were all fraternal, and were differentially treated by their parents.

RESEARCH DESIGN

Beginning with our initial family of quintuplets, we saw each cohort that was added to the sample from the age of three months and then every three months until the age of two years, at two and a half years, and then every year with measures that addressed the above hypotheses. We were able to see the children yearly from the age of two through age nine, and one family at age twelve. The initial measures were developmental and object relations measures: the Bayley mental and motor development scales, and the Décarie object relations and object constancy scales. The developmental tests were changed to adapt to their growing developmental status: the Stanford Binet,

Form L-M intelligence test from ages two or two and a half through age five, and the Wechsler Intelligence Scale for Children, Revised through age twelve. Personality measures were added as the children developed: the Rorschach Ink Blot Test and the Draw a Person Test from ages five through age twelve. The measures and administration methods will be more fully described in Chapter 4.

REFERENCES

Ablon, S. L., Harrison, A. M., Valenstein, A. F., and Gifford, S. 1986. Special Solutions to Phallic Aggressive Conflicts in Male Twins. *The Psychoanalytic Study of the Child.* 41, 239–257.

Ainslie, R. 1985. *The Psychology of Twinship*. Lincoln and London: The University of Nebraska Press.

Ainslie, R. C., Olmstead, K. M., & O'Laughlin, D. D. 1987. The early developmental context of twinship. Some limitations of the equal environmental hypothesis. *American Journal of Orthopsychiatry*, 57(1), 120–124.

Anderson, M. L. 1985. The mental health advantage of twinship. *Perspectives in Psychiatric Care*, 23(3), 114–116.

Athanassiou, C. 1986. A study of the vicissitudes of identification in twins. *International Journal of Psychoanalysis*, 67(3), 329–335.

Basit, A. 1972. Rorschach study of personality development in identical and fraternal twins. *Journal of Personality Assessment*, 36(1), 23–27.

Brooks, J., & Lewis, M. 1974. Attachment behavior in thirteen-month-old, opposite-sex twins. *Child Development*, 45(1), 243–247.

Cohen, D. J., Allen, M. G., Polin, W., Inoff, G., Werner, M., & Dibble, E. 1972. Personality development in twins. Competence in the newborn and pre-school periods. *American Academy of Child Psychiatry*, 11(4), 621–644.

Conway, D., Lytton, H., & Pysh, F. 1980. Twin-singleton language differences. *Canadian Journal of Behavioural Science*, 12(3), 264–271.

Dolan, A. B., & Matheny, A. P. 1978. A distinctive growth cure for a group of children with academic learning problems. *Journal of Learning Disabilities*, 1(8), 490–494.

Feinstein, S. 1985. Multiple Births and Twins. In H. I. Kaplan, & B. I. Sadock (Eds.) *Comprehensive Textbook of Psychiatry*. Baltimore, Maryland: Williams & Wilkins.

Goldberg, S., Perotta, M., Minde, K., & Carter, C. 1986. Maternal behavior and attachment in low birth-weight twins and singletons. *Child Development*, 57(1), 34–46.

Goshen-Gottstein, E. 1980. The Mothering of Twins, Triplets and Quadruplets. *Psychiatry*, 43, 189–204.

Hamilton, J., Blewett, D., & Sydiak, D. 1971. Ink blot responses of identical and fraternal twins. *Journal of Genetic Psychology*, 119(1), 37–41.

Hay, D. A., & O'Brien, P. J. Early Influences on the School Adjustment of Twins. 1987. *Acta Genet Med Gemeliol.* 36, 239–248.

Hay, D. A., Prior, M., Collett, S., and Williams, M. 1987. Speech and Language Development in Preschool Twins. *Acta Genet Med Gemeliol.* 36, 213–223.

Johnston, C., Prior, M., & Hay, D. 1984. Prediction of reading disability in twin boys. *Developmental Medicine and Child Neurology*, 26(5), 588–595.

Josepth, E. D. 1975. Psychoanalysis-science and research. Twin studies as a paradigm. *Journal of the American Psychoanalytic Association*, 23(1), 3–31.

Krall, V., Feinstein, S., & Kennedy, D. 1980. Birth weight and measures of development, object constancy, and attachment in multiple birth infants: A brief report. *International Journal of Behavioral Development*, 3, 501–505.

Matheny, A. P., Dolan, A. B., & Wilson, R. S. 1976. Twins with academic learning problems: Antecedent characteristics. *American Journal of Orthopsychiatry*, 46(3), 464–469.

Matheny, A. P., Wilson, R. S., Dolan, A. P., & Krantz, J. Z. 1982. Behavioral contrasts in twinships: Stability and patterns of differences in childhood. *Annual Progress in Child Psychiatry and Child Development*, 229–245.

Moilanen, I. 1987. Dominance and Submissiveness Between Twins I. Perinatal and Development Aspects. *Acta Genet Med Gemellol.* 36, 249–255.

Moilanen, I. 1987. Dominance and Submissiveness Between Twins II. Consequences for Mental Health. *Acta Genet Med Gemellol.* 36, 257–265.

Moilanen, I. 1988. Psychic Vulnerability as a Sequel to Perinatal Morbidity. *Acta Paediatrica Scandinavica.* Supplementum No. 344, 77, 95–105.

Paluszny, M., & Abelson, A. G. 1975. Twins in a child psychiatry clinic. *American Journal of Psychiatry*, 132(4), 434–436.

Rehmann, J. T. 1979. A study of the conjoint drawings of identical and fraternal twins: a pilot study. *Art Psychotherapy*, 6(2), 109–117.

Riese, M. L. 1980. Assessment of gestational age in twins: Lack of agreement among procedures. *Journal of Pediatric Psychology*, 5(1), 9–16.

Riese, M. L. 1983. Behavioral patterns in full-term and preterm twins. *Acta Geneticae Medicae et Gemellologiae: Twin Research*, 32(3–4), 209–220.

Riese, M. L. 1984. Within-pair differences in newborn twins: Effects of gender and gestational age on behavior. *Acta Geneticae Medicae et Gemellalogiae: Twin Research*, 33(2), 159–164.

Riese, M. L. 1988. Size for Gestational Age and Neonatal Temperament in Full-Term and Preterm AGA-SGA Twin Pairs. *Journal of Pediatric Psychology*, 13(4), 521–530.

Showers, J., & McCleery, J. T. 1984. Research on twins: implications for parenting. *Child Care, Health, and Development*, 10(6), 391–404.

Siemon, M. 1980. The separation-individuation process in adult twins. *American Journal of Psychotherapy*, 34(3), 387–400.

Sigman, & Parmalee, A. H. 1979. Longitudinal evaluation of the preterm infant. Chapter 10 in T. M. Field (Ed.), *Infants Born at Risk.* New York: S P Medical & Scientific Books.

Szajnberg, N. M., Skrinjaric, J., and Moore, A. 1989. Affect Attunement, Attachment, Temperament, and Zygosity: A Twin Study. *Journal of the American Academy of Child and Adolescent Psychiatry*, 28(2), 249–253.

Terry, G. E. 1975. The separation-individuation process in same-sex twins: A review of the literature. *Maternal-Child Nursing Journal.* 4(2), 121–128.

Tomasello, M., Mannic, S., & Kruger, A. C. 1986. Linguistic environment of 1- to 2-year-old twins. *Developmental Psychology*, 22(2), 169–176.

von Broembsen, F. 1988. The Twinship: A Paradigm Towards Separation and Integration. *The American Journal of Psychoanalysis*. 48(4), 355–365.
Wilson, R. S. 1974. Twins: Mental development in the preschool years. *Developmental Psychology*, 10(4), 580–588.
Wilson, R. S. 1985. Risk and resilience in early mental development. *Developmental Psychology*, 21(5), 795–805.
Wilson, R. S., & Matheny, A. P. 1983. Mental development: Family environment and genetic influences. *Intelligence*, 7(2), 195–215.

CHAPTER 2

Our Children

The subject cohorts were chosen as they presented themselves to us, and we had sufficient time to add them to our sample. It was on the basis of chance that each cohort was added to the sample, and sample size of the original set of five families was dictated by time considerations. We added three sets of triplets, that are not part of the basic sample. Triplets A were followed through two years; Triplets B were seen only at three months; Triplets C were seen at 9 years of age. These data are presented in some of the chapters for comparative purposes.

It is interesting to note that the range of birth weights and gestation (conception) ages forms a natural experiment, from lowest birth weights to highest, and earliest gestations to latest. Tables 2.1 and 2.2 show this.

The quintuplets ranged in birth weight from 767 to 1376 grams. Their gestation was 32 weeks in duration. They were in incubator between five and eight weeks, and hospital discharge was between six to eight weeks. Oxygen was administered from 12–36 hours. In our statistical comparisons, birth order was not found to have an effect, aside from its influence on birth weight, so it is not included in the tabular material. Note that these quints were small for date in comparison to the next cohort, the first set of quadruplets. This cohort was of mixed gender.

The first set of quadruplets ranged in birth weight from 1413 to 1889 grams. Gestation was 31 weeks. This cohort were in incubator from 11 days to three weeks, and were discharged from the hospital between two and three weeks. No oxygen was reported used. In this cohort there are three boys and one girl.

The second set of quadruplets ranged in birth weight from 1179 to 1932 grams and were 34 weeks in gestation. This is another cohort that was small for date. They were three to four weeks in incubator,

Table 2.1. Birth information about subjects

Cohorts	Birth Weight (gms)	Gestation	In Incubator	Hospital Discharge	Oxygen
Quintuplets	767–1378	32 weeks	5–8 weeks	6–8 weeks	12–36 hours
Quadruplets 1	1413–1889	31 weeks	11 days–3 weeks	2–3 weeks	None
Quadruplets 2	1179–1932	34 weeks	3–4 weeks	18 days–5 weeks	None
Triplets 1	2159–2301	36 weeks	Short time	5–10 days	None
Triplets 2	2528–2727	38 weeks	None	5 days	None
Triplets A	1989–2017	34 weeks	None	1–11 days	None
Triplets B	2528–2983	38 weeks	None	6 days	None
Triplets C	1932–2131	36 weeks	None	5 days	None

Table 2.2. Birthweights

Sex	Weight (gms)
Female	767
Male	923
Female	1335
Male	1378
Female	1378
Female	1413
Male	1577
Male	1861
Male	1889
Female	1179
Female	1534
Female	1619
Male	1932
Male	2301
Female	2301
Female	2159
Male	2727
Male	2642
Female	2528
Female	2017
Female	2003
Male	1989
Female	2983
Female	2642
Female	2528
Female	2131
Female	1989
Female	1932

and were discharged between 18 days and five weeks. One child, a male child, was retained because of hip dislocation. Oxygen was not used with these children. In this cohort, there are three girls, and one boy.

The first set of triplets, added at nine months of age to the study, ranged in birth weight from 2159 to 2301 grams and were 36 weeks in gestation. They were reported to be in incubators a "short time" (quote from the family). They were discharged from the hospital between five and 10 days. No oxygen was given to these children in the premature nursery. One girl child returned to the hospital as an infant for hernia surgery. In this cohort, there are two girls and one boy.

The second set of triplets ranged in birth age from 2528 to 2727 grams, and were 38 weeks in gestation. No time in the incubator was needed, they were returned from the hospital "right away" (parental quote), and oxygen was not needed. In this cohort, there are two boys and one girl.

All multiple births were the result of fertility drugs, and all infants are fraternal. For quadruplets set 2, the infants were second born, after a daughter aged five. A drug had been taken for menstrual irregularity, and this drug was believed to have acted as a fertility drug in this case also.

Three additional families of triplets will be referred to in the body of the manuscript. The first set of triplets (hereafter referred to as "Triplets A") were fertility induced fraternals, delivered by Cesarean section. They ranged in birth weight from 1989 to 2017 grams and were in hospital from one to 11 days. One boy child had merconium in his amniotic fluid and was watched in the special care unit for 24 hours. The day he was released, a staph infection of his right big toe was found, and he was placed on penicillin and stayed in the hospital an extra 10 days. These children were not in incubator, and they were of 34 weeks gestation. They were seen at 3, 11, and 15 months, and at two years. There are two girls and a boy in this cohort.

A second additional set of triplets, (hereafter referred to as "Triplets B"), were seen at three months. They ranged in birth weight from 2528 to 2983 grams, and were of 38 weeks gestation. There was no time in incubator or oxygen, and they were returned to the home "right away," at six days. These children were not the product of fertility drugs. They included a monozygotic pair of twins and a fraternal triplet. These girl triplets were delivered also by Cesarean section. There were two prior boy siblings, ages six and three.

As a result of some publicity in the newspaper, the parents of a set of identical girl triplets ("Triplets C"), genetically born, contacted us out of interest. The triplets were tested at nine years of age, and provide some comparison data for our fraternal triplets at age nine. The birth weights of these girls were between 1932 and 2131 grams. They were of 36 weeks gestation. They required no special hospital care and were discharged on time.

CHAPTER 3

The Families and How They Coped

The most frequent questions asked of our families have been: "How are you doing it?" and "How did you do it?" Needless to say, it is the first year that was the most difficult. Goshen-Gottstein (1980) reports that her mothers of multiples experienced the births as a shock and many with ambivalence. The demands for her families were greatest during the first year of life. She reports, however, that they came to relate warmly to their infants in a relatively short time. She also reported that there was more opportunity to adapt to the multiple birth when the infants came home separately. Her families belonged to the middle or lower socioeconomic class of families living in Israel.

Information concerning our cohorts comes from observations during the first year and from a brief questionnaire. A summary profile of our parents would describe them as college graduates between 25 and 35 years of age. The mothers ranged in age at the time of the birth of the multiples between 26 and 30 years of age. The fathers were between 27 and 34 years of age. The mothers remained home for most of the first year of life of the children with the exception of one mother who worked on Saturdays as a retail buyer of children's clothing. The fathers were in professional-managerial level positions, including a certified public accountant, lawyer, sales manager, and manufacturer's representative.

All the families bought new homes very shortly before or after the birth of the multiples to make room for their expanded needs. They were located in pleasant suburban surroundings, and there was ample room within and without for the children to grow and to flourish. Two of the families moved at preschool age of the children to other cities out of state. One family returned to the Chicago suburban area, and one family continues to reside outside of the state.

The parents waited between four and a half and six years after marriage to have the multiple birth; most waited six years. During the first year, various arrangements were made for caretaking functions in addition to the extensive involvement of both parents in the lives of these children. Two families had registered nurses, one for six months and one for the first year. All the others had some form of day help, and in addition, the extended families, most importantly the grandparents. For the quintuplets, there was always someone around the clock, and one or two in day help, in addition to the registered nurses. The families in Goshen-Gottstein's study also had baby nurses during the first year of life.

Characteristically, the fathers of our families engaged in caretaking activities during the time that they were at home. This included dressing, feeding, playing, taking for walks, bathing, reading—"loving . . . the works . . .," to quote one father. Another quote, from a mother: the father was a "wonderful support." The mothers were caretakers along with the above mentioned support systems.

Reports on special preferences of the infants for caretakers varied. Two families report that a maternal grandmother was a favorite. Two families report no special preferences. One family reported that a particular day helper became a special preference to all, after 18 months. For the first year, one might summarize that there were no special preferences reported for the parental figures. "They seemed to like every one." This is an interesting observation, given our concern about the effects of multiple caretaking on attachment.

The support systems included spouses, friends, professional help to varying extent, and their household help. Dr. Feinstein was available as a consultant to all the parents during the course of the study, and some consulted him more than others. Particular slumps occurred at about nine months in the lives of these families. It was usually at this time that Dr. Feinstein described a condition he called "battle fatigue," and he recommended time away from the children. Most parents were able to take some time off, even if it was to do other chores. They managed to be away from the children on the average of one night a week. One parent managed this by having an outside sitter one day a week. Some were able to manage a vacation within a six month period. Goshen-Gottstein reported that the mothers of her cohorts often spent time away from the infants for doctors appointments or shopping. We encouraged needed rest periods and/or vacations for parental mental health.

The family stresses were great during this first year. Some of them were: "Financial has been continual; marital because the parents didn't have time for each other, only for the task at hand . . . must make time together away from the children, must get away regularly, i.e. every six months minimum." "Physical, the pressure you're most aware of and in the long run the easiest to cope with." "Physical stress stemmed from the constant care demanded by the children." "Utter exhaustion the first six months." The comment most revealing about these families and seems to characterize our observations of them is the following from a mother: "and I developed a tremendous understanding for each other's needs, so the emotional stress was certainly lessened. . . . I really forget a lot about the first year."

These are families with many outside interests and rich inner resources which undoubtedly enabled them to cope better with the stress. Hobbies reported by the mothers were: photography, reading, jogging, golf, skiing, tennis, quilting, sewing, needlework, community activities, cooking, and exercise. The father's interests included skiing, jogging, swimming, golf, tennis, reading, running, racquet ball, photography, music, and exercise.

ADDITIONAL FAMILIES

The additional families were very comparable to the original sample in sociocultural and educational variables. The parents are college graduates or more, and the parental occupations are professional-managerial. The age of the mothers at the multiple birth were between 29 and 34. For these sets of triplets, one of the mothers chose to continue working and placed the triplets in day care. This particular family reported that the children were much attached to the day care personnel, but these parents also found time to play and to relate to them. Another family had live in help for the first six months, and a mother-in-law visited for two months. Another family had grandmothers live in for one month each. Babysitters were also utilized. Parents in these cohorts also shared care taking and play experiences with each other. These cohorts also indicate considerable support from spouses, friends, neighbours, professional contacts at our hospital, and the day care facility mentioned. The stresses were described very similarly to the cohorts in the nuclear sample.

SAMPLE QUOTES

Cohort A

"The biggest stress was emotional exhaustion. Some nights I couldn't stand holding the kids any longer. They woke each other up at night and we got very little sleep. The most difficult times were when the kids got sick. They either got sick at the same time or in close sequence, giving us little time to recover our own strength. While we were conscious of how much money we were spending, we didn't have too much stress due to financial matters. We did skimp on getting 'help'. If I had to do it over, I'd hire baby sitters at dinner hours every night. And I'd try to get out alone one night a week. In general, we did not have time to feel 'marital stress'." This family also reported some difference of opinion as to whether to let the children cry, a frequent difference of opinion among parents of singleton children.

Cohort B

"The financial stress was enormous. Our house was too small." This family has two older sons, and the birth was not from fertility drugs. "The babies' birth was not covered by insurance, formula and diaper costs outrageous. Day care is extremely expensive, but mother must work to keep her sanity. Finding time for ourselves is difficult, but we work at it. The babies are very good and delightful." This was written when the infants were age one year.

Cohort C

This cohort had an 18½ month old daughter when their identical girl triplets were born. They had the live in help of mother and mother-in-law each for a month. They had very little additional support. Friends helped only occasionally, and there was no professional help. They report little time for themselves or social life during that first year. This quote from the father tells the story: "Started new business, limited income . . . for about a few years. No support systems. Very overwhelming and trying period."

If one might make a comparison between these cohorts and the nuclear sample, and between cohorts A and C, and B, one might read between the lines that cohort B mother was less stressed by the emotional and exhaustion stresses because she gets out of the house to work. She seemed to remember getting more enjoyment from the children during that first year: "What a rewarding experience. We're still fascinated with them." Our other mothers also enjoyed their children. We are also not suggesting that mothers of multiples go back to work immediately. The consensus of most of the reactions concerning the first year, however, is that making time for mother away from the children during the day and time for the social life for both parents away from the children can play an important role towards reducing the stress of that first year.

REFERENCES

Goshen-Gottstein, E. (1980) The Mothering of Twins, Triplets, and Quadruplets. *Psychiatry*, 43, 189–204.

CHAPTER 4

Observing How They Grew

This study is a small sample study of the original five families and nineteen children; and three families of triplets added later for comparative purposes. Although this is a small sample, its advantage is that we have longitudinal measures over a nine year period for all subjects and over twelve years for one family.

Our initial hypotheses concerned development and attachment (Krall, Feinstein, & Kennedy, 1980). We chose the most current and reliable developmental and affective tests available in 1973 when the study was initiated. As the children matured, we changed to measures more appropriate to their developmental ages for cognition, and incorporated tests of language and personality.

MEASURES OF THE FIRST PHASE OF THE STUDY: 3–24 MONTHS

Bayley Infant Scales of Mental and Motor Development

The Bayley Scales (Bayley, 1969) provide mental and motor developmental indices of developmental age and developmental quotient. We did not have a control sample as multiple births are a rare event. Our sample was compared with the Bayley normative sample for each age being studied. The Bayley continues to 30 months. We administered the Bayley mental and motor scales from three months through 18 months every three months and at 24 months. In certain instances mentioned in the text we also administered the mental and motor scales at 21 months and the mental scale at 30 months for two very low birth weight children. We did not administer the motor scale past 24 months because we did not have the physical equipment for the motor scales in the home environment. We did improvise at times by having the children walk up and down their own stairs.

The Bayley scales were administered in each family's home. Most of the families moved shortly before or after the multiple birth and the homes afforded excellent physical environments for test administration. We used the children's own bassinettes and later their own high chairs for the testing. The children were always in the comfort and support of their own physical surroundings. The mother was always present during the testing, and the mother chose the child to be tested first in the early infancy stage. Later the children were asked to choose who would be tested first.

The Bayley was always administered sequentially to each child separately by two examiners and the mother assisting in the examination. Any item requiring physical handling was administered by the mother with careful instructions from the examiners. Each examiner followed a particular child wherever possible. The second examiner was then the recorder for that child. The primary examiner would report the pass-fail to the recorder. There was seldom a disagreement, but if there was there was quick resolution of the pass-fail. Each examiner then scored his own examinations. From age two on the primary examiner administered the examination to each of his children alone and the two examiners could test simultaneously.

We had thought initially that the mothers might be upset at the reporting of pass-fail in their presence. On the contrary, our mothers were very gratified to see how much their infants could do and often commented upon this. Occasionally they would say that a child had done something for them that was a fail during the examination. They understood our explanation that it probably was an accomplishment that was emerging and not yet stable.

The scores for the Bayley were obtained for Birth Age and then adjusted for gestation. The method of computing gestation or conception age scores followed the method reported by Hunt and Rhodes (1977) and is described in detail in their article. A more complete discussion concerning the pros and cons of using an age correction for prematurity will be discussed in the chapter on development and prematurity.

Décarie Scales of Objectal Development and Object Constancy

The Décarie Scales of Objectal development and Object Constancy (Décarie, 1965) provide criterion measures with equivalent norms in mental age. The Objectal scale measures such criteria as searching for the breast at two months to such more sophisticated abilities as discriminating mother's pleasurable and unpleasurable reaction at 12–15 months. Some adjustments were made for ordinal reliability and validity.

The mental age scores were used for statistical purposes. When there was a range of months for a particular test item, such as 12–15 months, the lower month level was used for criterion a for the item, and the higher month level was used for criterion b for items that had two scoring levels. This provided a continuous ordinal scale and greatly increased the statistical usefulness of this scale.

The first criterion for the Object Constancy scale concerns whether the three-month old infant can follow a dropped ball, and later criterion measures determine whether a child can follow a moving object under one to several screens with visible and invisible displacements to 18–20 months. The age range problem for a particular criterion was handled similarly to the Objectal Scale. Where there were two parts to the criterion level, the lower mental age was assigned to item a and the higher mental age was assigned to item b.

The order of the examination for each infant during this phase of the study was Bayley mental scale, Bayley motor scale, and the Décarie scales. This sequence was followed with each infant as much as possible. Occasionally an infant would become fretful and we would discontinue testing with that infant for the time being and return at the end of the testing session to complete the examination on that infant. While one infant was being tested the others were with a caretaker in another room and in another part of the home.

Behavior measures were noted by the recording examiner and incorporated into the reports written after each session. The testings were usually done in one day, but in the early infancy of the quintuplets, we did make two visits per testing. The findings were shared informally with the mother at the end of each testing session. At the end of our individual scoring procedures each examiner reviewed his findings and the behaviors that accompanied his findings and wrote a brief report. This brief report became part of the research data base. It was also sent to the parents for themselves and their pediatrician if so desired.

In the tables which will follow the results chapters you will note some changes in numbers of subjects from testing to testing. One family of triplets did not join the project until nine months of age and then only for the Décarie measures. The N for three and six months is 16 instead of 19. At age nine months the N is 12 for the

Bayley measures because this set of triplets and one set of quadruplets were not tested, the latter due to snow. There was also inability to obtain data for the Motor Scale and Décarie scales for particular infants on a particularly stressful day: 24 months for the Motor Scale, and 18 and 24 months on the Décarie Scales.

MEASURES USED FOR THE SECOND PHASE OF THE STUDY: 30 MONTHS TO 7 YEARS

Human Figure Drawings

Beginning at 30 months of age, each child was asked to draw a picture of a person. If a boy was drawn first, the child was asked to draw a girl; if a girl was drawn first, the child was asked to draw a boy. These drawings were scored according to the Harris revision of the Goodenough method (Harris, 1963). This method of scoring is attentive to detail and proportions of the figures. The raw scores of details and proportions yields a developmental Standard Score with a mean of 100 and a standard deviation of 15, obtained from separate tables for boys and girls.

The Stanford Binet, Form L-M Intelligence Test

The Stanford Binet, Form L-M Intelligence Test was administered between two and a half and five years of age. For the later term birth infants the Binet could be administered at age two. This means that some of the infants had the Bayley at two and some the Binet. The Binet is a mental age scale. Between ages two and five and a half, the age span for each mental age level is six months and each item is given one month's credit. The score is in mental age and intelligence quotient. The latter may be obtained from a table using the chronological age and the mental age to obtain the IQ (Terman & Merrill, 1973). The standardization mean is an IQ of 100 with a standard deviation of 16.

Rorschach Ink Blot Test

The Rorschach Ink Blot test was administered to all children from ages five through nine. Later in the project, we administered the Rorschach from ages three on. Prior to age nine the method was a standard administration with the exception that the inquiry was obtained after each card. This was to avoid the loss of responses due to the faulty memory of preschool children and an increase in their restlessness. From age nine the administration was entirely standard. All protocols were scored according to the Exner Comprehensive system (Exner & Weiner, 1982). In addition, all human and quasi-human responses were scored and evaluated with two scales: the Pruitt and Spilka scale (Pruitt & Spilka, 1964), and the Blatt Object Representation Scale (Blatt, 1976).

The Pruitt and Spilka scale (1964) gives weighted scores for all percepts from animals in human like activity to those with mythological content; human content with or without sex specified and in present or distant context; and human movement responses similarly scored: sex specified or unspecified and in present or distant context. The weights are from a scale of 1 to 18, the highest score of 18 being for human movement responses with sex specified and in present temporal context.

The Blatt Scale of Object Representations (1976) measures the differentiation, accuracy, level of integration, motivation, congruence of action, affective benevolence or malevolence, and activity level of the human or quasi-human responses on the Rorschach. There is no quantitative score assigned to these measures. A qualitative study of the responses, however, gives one an understanding of the object level of the responses in a given record.

Language Measure

The measure of language development at age two and a half was based on Valett's profile (Valett, 1965) of the Stanford Binet, L-M Intelligence Scale. All items of Comprehension for receptive speech and Vocabulary for expressive speech were accumulated to provide a total score of language development. The language measures were correlated with the Kohen-Raz Scales (1967) of the Bayley Infant Development Scales.

The Kohen-Raz monograph (1967) develops subscales from the Bayley Mental Scales that span the age range 2.9 months through 19.1 months. The scales include an Eye-Hand Scale, Manipulative Scale, Object Relations Scale, Imitation and Comprehension Scale, and Vocalization-Social Contact-Active Vocabulary Scale. The scales give a separate score for each age and each scale that can be compared with the language score and with the other scores of the Bayley, the Binet, and the human figure drawings.

MEASURES USED FOR THE THIRD PHASE OF THE STUDY: 7–9 YEARS

Human Figure Drawings

Described above.

Wechsler Intelligence Scale for Children, Revised

The Wechsler Intelligence Scale for Children, Revised (1974) was administered to all children at age seven, one family at age eight, and four families at age nine from the nuclear sample. An additional comparative sample of identical triplet girls was given the WISC-R at age nine. The WISC-R was designed for children between six and 16 years. The standardization provides a mean of 100 and a standard deviation of 15. The subtests we included in our test administration were Information, Similarities, Arithmetic, Vocabulary, and Comprehension from the Verbal Scale; and Picture Completion, Picture Arrangement, Block Design, Object Assembly, and Coding from the Performance Scale. The Digit Span and Maze tests were omitted because of time considerations. The WISC-R yields a Verbal IQ, a Performance IQ and a Full Scale IQ.

Rorschach Ink Blot Test

Described above.

ADDITIONAL TESTS FOR SPECIAL PROBLEMS

Beery Buktenika Visual Motor Integration Test

This is a visual motor drawing test comprised of designs of increasing difficulty that spans the ages from two to 15 with a scoring system that gives a mental age. Test norms were derived in 1964 and revised in 1982 (Beery, 1982).

Thematic Apperception Test

For some of the special problems, selected story telling cards of the Thematic Apperception Test (TAT) (Murray, 1943) were administered to elicit particular dynamics that were occurring at the time of referral. This was always during a regularly scheduled research visit.

GENERAL ADMINISTRATION METHODOLOGY

All children were tested within two weeks of their birthday, and never more than four weeks from their birthday at the later ages. Children were testing beginning at three months, and at regular intervals of three months through 18 months; two low birthweight children at 21 months; 24 and 30 months; three years; four years; five years; seven years; one family was tested at eight years; all but the latter family were tested at nine years. There was a followup testing on one family at twelve years.

Afte the age of three several of the families came to the clinic for testing. They came for one or two sessions and the siblings waited in the waiting room of the clinic or walked on the campus of the hospital while their siblings were being tested. They found this an enjoyable visit. This also allowed several of the families to have special issues addressed when there were particular problems they wished evaluated at the older school ages. For some of these testings that addressed particular emotional or school academic problems additional tests could be administered in the comfort of the clinic office and with more time to spare.

REFERENCES

Bayley, N. (1969). *Manual for the Bayley Scales of Infant Development*. New York: The Psychological Corporation.

Beery, K. E. (1982). *Revised Administration, Scoring, and Teaching Manual for the Developmental Test of Visual-Motor Integration*. Chicago, Illinois: Follett Publishing Company.

Blatt, S. J. (1976). *Clinical application of the assessment of the concept of the object on the Rorschach*. Unpublished manual.

Décarie, T. C. (1965). *Intelligence and affectivity in early childhood*. New York: International Universities Press.

Exner, J. E. Jr., & Weiner, I. B. (1982) *The Rorschach: A Comprehensive System. Volume 3. Assessment of Children and Adolescents*. New York: John Wiley & Sons.

Harris, D. B. 1963). *Children's Drawings as Measures of Intellectual Maturity*. New York: Harcourt, Brace & World, Inc.

Hunt, J. McV. & Užgiris, I. (1975) *Assessment of Infancy*. Urbana: University of Illinois Press.

Hunt, J. B., & Rhodes, L. (1977) Mental development of pre-term infants during the first year. *Child Development, 48*, 204–210.

Kohen-Rax, R. (1967). Scalogram analysis of some developmental sequences of infant behavior as measured by the Bayley Infant Scale of mental development. *Genetic Psychology Monographs, 76*, 3–21.

Murray, H. A. (1943). *Thematic Apperception Test Manual*. Cambridge, Massachusetts: Harvard University Printing Office.

Pruitt, W. A., & Spilka, B. (1964). Rorschach empathy-object relationship scale. *Journal of projective techniques and personality assessment, 28*, 331–336.

Teman, L. M., & Merrill, M. A. (1973). *Stanford-Binet Intelligence Scale*. Boston: Houghton Mifflin Company.

Wechsler, D. (1974). *Wechsler Intelligence Scale for Children, Revised*. New York: The Psychological Corporation.

CHAPTER 5

"Catch Up" by Two Years of Age

Reviews of the literature on prematurity and low birth weight (Holmes, Reich, & Pasternak, 1984; Kopp & Krakow, 1983) indicate a high relationship between birth weight as an effect of prematurity, and developmental outcome in high risk infants. The question has been raised as to whether there is continuity of developmental risk factors, or whether there is an all or none effect (Sigman, Cohen, & Forsythe, 1981). The answer seems to be that declining birth weight in association with perinatal complications results in handicap, and the greater the number of these factors, the poorer the developmental outcome (Sigman, & Parmalee, 1979).

Neligan, Kalvin, Scott, & Garside (1976) studied a comparative sample of those children that were of early gestation with those that were small for date and concluded that "those who were born too soon were at a meaningful advantage in their later development in comparison with those who were born too small". However, recent literature has demonstrated the importance of differentiating children with specific medical complications when discussing the outcome of prematures (Landry, Chapieski, Fletcher, & Demnson, 1988), and other research has demonstrated that some neurologically impaired preterms make recovery with or without remediation (Piper, Mazer, Silver, & Ramsay, 1988).

Greenberg & Crnic (1988) have demonstated that for their sample of preterm and full term children there were no differences between them at 24 months corrected age with the exception of motor development, on a wide range of measures, including mental development, expressive and receptive language skills.

This is a complex area of investigation, with many variables impacting on development. Our sample (refer again to Table 1.1) includes four families that were of less than 38 weeks gestation; and three families that were small for date. At least half the sample were below 1500 grams. The sample, if one studies the birth weights in Table 1.1, are on a continuum for birth weight.

The question of whether to correct for prematurity continues to plague the literature (Holmes, Reich, & Pasternak, 1984; Siegel, 1983). The current conclusion from Siegel (1983) is that it is important under a year, with significant differences for the premature children studied, but beyond that it does not produce significant effects. The correction factor may obscure early deficiencies that later emerge (Caputo, Goldstein, & Taub, 1979). We have been particularly concerned with difficulties that may emerge at school age, to be addressed in a later chapter.

Our first data presentations will deal with the question of apparent "catch up" in the premature, when adjusted and unadjusted scores are used; and the relationship of early developmental scores to birth weight. We will be interested in whether there is a relationship of developmental scores to birth weight; and whether there is a point at which birth weight effects are diminished. Later chapters will deal with whether there are prematurity effects on later abilities, such as language and school functioning.

RESULTS

Adjusted and Unadjusted Developmental Scores

Bayley (MDI) and Motor (PDI) scores, adjusted for gestation and smoothed according to the method reported by Hunt and Rhodes (1977), fall within one standard deviation of the mean of the scale (100) at each age interval tested beyond six months through 24 months of age. They are higher than one standard deviation at 30 months and 36 months. Smoothed adjusted mean motor scores were above one standard deviation at three months. Raw score gain appeared relatively constant from 12 months on, with highest MDI adjusted scores achieved at 36 months (Mean, 129). In this sample, MDI is higher than PDI from six months on (Tables 5.1–5.4).

In contrast, there is a lag in both mental and motor development when unadjusted scores alone are observed, with apparent "catch up" occurring between 15 months and two years. Measures go beyond normative development and appear to approach socioeconomic and educational level expectancy by three years. Adjusted MDI mean mental score is 129 and unadjusted MDI score is 125 at three years.

Table 5.1. Correlation of unadjusted age mean scores for mental development with birth weight

Age in Months	3	6	9	12	15	18		24	30	36
							Bayley/Binet			
N	16	16	12	19	19	19	9	10	19	19
Correlations	.85	.92	.93	.82	.83	.86	.17	.72	.79	.49
Mean MDI	86	81	79	82	95	98	88	129	120	125
Standard Deviations	11.6	26.9	25.2	25.0	27.4	28.8	5.1	13.3	21.2	13.9
p: Significant at Probability Level	.01	.01	.01	.01	.01	.01	.10	.02	.01	.05

Table 5.2. Correlation of smoothed adjusted age mean scores for mental development with birth weight

Age in Months	3	6	9	12	15	18		24	30	36
						Bayley/Binet				
N	16	16	12	19	19	19	9	10	19	19
Correlations	.64	.57	.78	.73	.80	.84	.09	.47	.72	.35
Mean MDI	115	115	98	100	106	109	95	135	126	129
Standard Deviations	16.1	17.6	18.9	18.3	23.0	22.2	5.9	7.4	22.0	13.8
p: Significant at Probability Level	.05	.05	.01	.01	.01	.01	.10	.10	.01	NS

Table 5.3. Correlation of unadjusted mean scores for motor development with birth weight

Age in Months	3	6	9	12	15	18	24
N	16	16	12	19	19	19	13
Correlations	.14	.72	.95	.72	.84	.90	.56
Mean PDI	102	79	76	80	89	93	94
Standard Deviations	15.8	14.8	26.6	18.1	14.6	19.9	12.5
p: Significant at Probability Level	NS	.01	.01	.01	.01	.01	.05

Table 5.4. Correlation of smoothed adjusted age mean scores for motor development with birth weight

Age in Months	3	6	9	12	15	18	24
N	16	16	12	19	19	19	13
Correlations	−.10	−.06	.88	.42	.69	.86	.60
Mean PDI	130	111	97	98	96	101	101
Standard Deviations	20.0	21.8	19.0	20.2	13.5	16.0	13.6
p: Significant at Probability Level	NS	NS	.01	NS	.01	.01	.05

Correlations with Birth Weight

Adjusted MDI scores were significantly correlated with birth weight from three months through 30 months. Adjusted PDI scores were significantly correlated with birth weight at 9, 15, 18, and 24 months. Unadjusted correlations followed a similar pattern. Higher birth weight children tended to receive higher scores on both scales during this period.

Mental and Motor Development Over Time

Tables 5.5, 5.6, 5.7, and 5.8 show the average, above average, and below average mental and motor development for unadjusted and adjusted scores from three months to three years for mental development and from three months to two years for motor development.

Both adjusted and unadjusted scores of mental development show gradual increase of average and above average scores, with most children demonstrating above average scores by 36 months. It is

Table 5.5. Average, above average, and below average unadjusted mental scores

Age in Months	3	6	9	12	15	18	24	30	36
N	16	16	12	19	19	19	19	19	19
Below 90	11	12	9	11	8	8	7	0	1
90–100	2	1	0	3	2	2	2	4	0
Above 100	3	3	3	5	9	9	10	15	18

Table 5.6. Average, above average, and below average adjusted mental scores

Age in Months	3	6	9	12	15	18	24	30	36
N	16	16	12	19	19	19	19	19	19
Below 90	1	0	4	7	5	5	2	0	1
90–100	2	4	3	2	2	2	6	2	0
Above 100	13	12	5	10	12	12	11	17	18

Table 5.7. Average, above average, and below average unadjusted motor scores

Age in Months	3	6	9	12	15	18	24
N	16	16	12	19	19	19	13
Below 90	4	11	9	12	9	10	5
90–100	1	5	0	5	6	2	3
Above 100	11	0	3	2	4	7	5

Table 5.8. Average, above average, and below average adjusted motor scores

Age in Months	3	6	9	12	15	18	24
N	16	16	12	19	19	19	13
Below 90	1	2	4	4	4	4	2
90–100	1	5	1	6	6	6	4
Above 100	14	9	7	9	9	9	7

interesting to note, however, that the children who lagged behind until 30 months were from two low birth weight cohorts.

This dramatic demonstraation is not true for the motor development scores. Even until 24 months, the last age they were tested for motor development, there were ten children with below average unadjusted motor scores and four children with below average adjusted motor development scores.

DISCUSSION

The results suggest that these low birth weight, preterm multiple birth infants lagged behind in development during the first two years when scored according to birth age (unadjusted scores). When unadjusted scores are used, there is an apparent acceleration in score and "catch up" by 15 months to two years, as suggesteda by Hunt and Rhodes (1977). When measures are adjusted for prematurity, mental and motor scores are in the average range or above. Unadjusted scores showed positive acceleration with age, and appear to catch up at 15 months for mental scores and at 18 months for motor scores. Scores continued to increase until the average mental score was 125 for unadjusted and 129 for adjusted measures at three years of age. Comparable motor scores were not obtained past two years.

The above average adjusted scores at three months and at six months may reflect some overcorrection of scores for prematurity, as suggested by Hunt and Rhodes (1977). There may also be artifacts in the scales at that age, and/or the advantage of increased extrauterine experiences associated with prematurity, which diminish during the second half of the first year. The increases in score past two years may reflect the increased socialization experiences of their high socioeconomic status.

There has been recent concern that correction for gestation ignores specific high risk factors that are apart from low birth weight itself, that interfere with later development (Caputo, Goldstein, & Taub, 1981). Landry (1984) suggests that corrected Bayley scores at six and

12 months are deceptive, and may obscure the need for early intervention. Siegel (1983) reports that the use of a correction for degree of prematurity may be appropriate for the early months, but in most cases at one year and after, there were no significant differences between the predictive ability of the corrected and uncorrected scores. We will be interested in our long term follow up data in later chapters to determine whether there are high risk effects that later emerge in the developmental data.

We found a relationship between birth weight and developmental status. There were strong correlations with birth weight for mental development, for both adjusted and unadjusted scores. Benton (1940), an early reviewer, did not note such a relationship. Campbell (personal report) did not find significant correlations between birth weight and scores on the Bayley in their work with twins. Wilson (1978) did find such a relationship at selected ages. Our findings may relate to the wide range of birth weights, from 767 to 2727 grams; and/or to the larger multiple status of our children. There did seem to be such a relationship when our small for date infants are compared with our appropriate for date infants. Heavier, but more premature quads received higher test scores than lighter, but less premature quints throughout the first two years. The possibility of intrauterine malnourishment or deprivation due to crowding and greater number among the latter is one hypothesis that could account for such differences. It is also possible that birth weight itself is a complex variable that is correlated with prenatal malnutrition and/or subsequent complications. A further hypothesis is that differential behavioral characteristics may be observed, and that patterns of parent-child interactions may differ. Having multiple children may greatly affect parental interaction with these children, as has been observed by Goshen-Gottstein (1980).

Our adjusted Bayley mental development index of 116 and unadjusted Bayley mental developmental index of 110 agree well with Sigman and Parmalee's (1979) Bayley score of 113 for their high socioeconomic English speaking prematures at two years of age. Birth weight in our sample is no longer related to mental development at 36 months; and the scores obtained beyond two years of age seem to be more related to socioeconomic effects. Recent studies of the premature have pointed to the primacy of environment, socioeconomic, and caretaking effects on the later development of prematures. Hunt (1981) reports that "socio-educational influences may have overwhelmed and obscured associations with major biological variables by early childhood." Sigman, Cohen, Beckwith, and Parmalee (1981) indicate that the influence of preterm birth is modulated by familial influences in the first 18 months, and additionally, by sociocultural variables in the succeeding year.

A final comment might be addressed to the motor index scores, which lagged behind the mental scores, except for the three month inflated measures. Both Holmes (1984) and Siegel (1982) have commented on this finding for premature infants. The explanations they have suggested have been: 1. We may be more successful in evaluating motor delays with our knowledge of motor skills and our present measurement instruments. 2. Motor development may be more sensitive to brain damage effects at these early years; and 3. The small and weak prematures may have less opportunity for exercise in the early months, particularly if they remained in the intensive care nursery for any time. Ruff, McCarton, Kurtzberg, and Vaughan (1984) have demonstrated that high risk preterms show less rotating, fingering and transferring. They speculate that this could have an effect on learning about objects and later consequences for categorical learning, recognition memory, and later language development. It also might be noted that it was not always the lowest birth weight child who showed the most delay developmentally or the one who was later identified as the one having later academic difficulty. We shall explore some of these ideas in later chapters.

REFERENCES

Benton, A. L. (1980). Mental Development of Prematurely Born Children. *American Journal of Orthopsychiatry*, 10, 719–746.

Caputo, D. V., Goldstein, K. E., & Taub, H. B. (1981). Neonatal compromise and later psychological development. A 10-year longitudinal study. In. S. L. Friedman & E. Sigman (Eds.), *Preterm Birth and Psychological Development*. New York: Academic Press.

Goshen-Gottstein, E. R. (1980). The mothering of twins, triplets, and quadruplets. *Psychiatry*, 43, 189–204.

Greenberg, M. T., & Crnic, K. A. (1988). Longitudinal Predictors of Developmental Status and Social Interaction in Premature and Full-Term Infants at Age Two. *Child Development*, 59, 554–570.

Holmes, D. L., Reich, J. H., & Pasternak, J. F. (1984). The High Risk Infant Beyond the Neonatal Period. In D. L. Holmes, J. N. Reich, & J. F. Pasternak (Eds.) *The Development of Infants Born at Risk*. Hillsdale, New Jersey: Lawrence Erlbaum Associates, Publishers.

Hunt, J. V. (1981). Predicting intellectual disorders in childhood for preterm infants with birthweights below 1501 gm. In S. L. Friedman & M. Sigman (Eds.), *Preterm Birth and Psychological Development*. New York: Academic Press.

Hunt, J. V., & Rhodes, L. (1977). Mental development of preterm infants during the first year. *Child Development*, 48, 204–210.

Kopp, C. B., & Krakow, J. B. (1983). The Developmentalist and the Study of Biological Risk: A view of the past with an eye toward the future. *Child Development*, 54, 1086–1109.

Landry, S. H., Fletcher, J. N., & Zarling, C. L. (1984). Differential outcomes associated with early medical complications in premature infants. *Journal of Pediatric Psychology*, 9, 386–399.

Landry, S. H., Chapieski, L., Fletcher, J. M., & Denson, S. (1988). Three Year Outcomes for Low Birth Weight Infants: Differential Effects of Early Medical Complications. *Journal of Pediatric Psychology*, 13, 317–328.

Neligan, G. A., Kalvin, I., Scott, M. D., & Garsiade, R. F. (1976). Born too soon or born too small. Follow-up study to seven years of age. London: William Heineman Medical Books Ltd.

Piper, M. C., Mazer, B., Silver, K. M., & Ramsay, M. (1988). Resolution of neurological symptoms in high-risk infants during the first two years of life. *Developmental Medicine and Child Neurology*, 30, 26–36.

Ruff, H. A., Mc Carton, C., Kurtzberg, D., & Vaughan Jr. H. G. (1984). Preterm infants' manipulative exploration of objects. *Child Development*, 55, 1166–1174.

Siegel, L. S. (1983). Correction for prematurity and its consequences for the assessment of the very low birth weight infant. *Child Development*, 54, 1176–1189.

Siegel, L. S., Saigal, S., Rosenbaum, P., Norton, R. A., Young, A., Berenbaum, S., & Stoskopf, B. (1982). Predictors of development in preterm and full-term infants. A model for detecting the 'at risk' child. *Journal of Pediatric Psychology*, 7, 135–149.

Sigman, M., Cohen, S. E., Beckwith, L., & Parmalee, A. H. (1981). Social and familial influences on the development of preterm infants. *Journal of Pediatric Psychology*, 6, 1–13.

Sigman, M., Cohen, S. E., & Forsythe, A. B. (1981). The Relation of Early Infant Measures to Later Development. In S. L. Friedman & M. Sigman (Eds.), *Preterm Birth and Psychological Development*. New York: Academic Press.

Sigman, M., & Parmalee, A. H. (1979). Longitudinal evaluation of the preterm infant. Chapter 10, in T. M. Field (Ed.), *Infants Born at Risk*. New York: S P Medical & Scientific Books.

Ungerer, J. A., & Sigman, M. (1983). Developmental lags in preterm infants from one to three years of age. *Child Development*, 54, 1217–1229.

Wilson, R. S. (1978). Synchronies in Mental Development: An epigenetic perspective. *Science*, 202, 939–948.

CHAPTER 6

Six Children and How They Grew

In this chapter, we will describe six children and their development from three months to three years of age. A girl and a boy were selected from low birth weight, middle birth weight, and higher birth weight cohorts as examples of the original sample of 19 infants. These examples may answer some of our questions concerning relative influence of birth weight versus other perinatal and prenatal factors of development; as well as the influence of the enriched social environment of our sample on development. A recent study demonstrates individual stability of behaviors in preterms as early as three months (Korner, Brown Jr., Byron, Dimiceli, Forrest, Stevenson, Lane, Constantinou, & Thom, 1989).

Each vignette includes some description of the child at each age level tested from three months through three years; the mental and motor developmental progression; objectal and object constancy development; and at three years, personality functioning as measured by the Rorschach and human figure drawings, where included.

VIGNETTES

Low Birth Weight Examples

Girl, A. This girl was the lowest in birth weight in her cohort. She is described in the three month report: "In spite of A.'s low birth weight and long stay in the hospital, she is comparing well with the other infants. There is some unevenness in sensory development, she visually recognizes the mother and vocalizes, but there is no social smile. . . . Motorically, she is slightly behind the other infants. She can balance her head, but is not turning over." There was no object constancy measure. Objectally, she could seek for the breast, but had not attained a social smile to mother or stranger. This was our baseline report for two months and 26 days. It will be most interesting to see how this child grew and developed over the first three years of life. At this time, her scores were mostly at the second month of life, both mentally and motorically, but normative for gestation age.

At six months, A. was functioning at the fifth month of development. She could grasp an object placed in her hand, and bang objects, and she was interested in sound production. She was not reaching for objects. Motorically, her hands were open, she sat with slight support, and her head was balanced. She could pull to a sitting position, and there were some progressive movements. She had not moved in object constancy, but there was a smiling response to both mother and examiner.

At nine months, there was little change in mental and motor development beyond the fifth month level. The major increments were the ability to grasp and retain objects (string, two of three cubes), attention to scribbling, and interest and ability to produce sound (rings bell purposively). Motorically, she could prehend a cube with partial thumb opposition, could turn from her back to her stomach, and from back to side. Object constancy had also begun to emerge; she could follow the falling ball from her left side. She could also discriminate mother from stranger, and smiled only at the talking and silent mother, and could be quieted by mother, in her presence.

At one year, A. was functioning at approximately the eighth month level of mental development. The developmental lag at this age was four months, as compared to two to three months for the heavier infants in this cohort. She appeared less alert than the other infants, as she was tested during her usual nap time. However, the other infants were also tested during nap time and appeared to be more alert. She was unable to grasp two cubes; however, purposive reaching seemed to be developing as she now secured the ring. There was increased visual perceptual interest and ability. She attended to scribbling, gave a playful response to the mirror, and looked at the picture book. She did not ring the bell, but was reported to listen selectively to words and to say da-da. She was also reported to jabber expressively, and to repeat a performance laughed at. Motorically, A. showed complete thumb opposition, but she did not as yet scoop a pellet. She could transfer objects, and there was pre-walking progression. She could sit alone, and could pull to standing, stand with support, and make stepping movements. Object constancy was at the 8–10 month level. She actively searched for and secured visually displaced objects (ball, pencil, stopwatch). Objectally, she achieved the nine month level: she responded positively to mother's play, negatively to its interruption, and negatively when a toy was taken away.

At 15 months, A. was functioning at the 11 month level of mental development and the 12 month level in motor development. She again appeared less responsive than the other girls, although this time she seemed more shy than sleepy. She could retain two cubes, and reached for the third. She looked for the contents of a box and uncovered the box. She could ring the bell and dangled a ring by its string. She could scribble and hold a crayon adaptively. Social behavior and verbal expression had advanced over the past three months. She cooperated in games, inhibited on command, and responded to a verbal request. She imitated words, and could say two words, her highest pass, at 14 months. The biggest gains occurred in fine and gross motor development, and seemed to be catching up to the others in the cohort in this regard. She now had a neat pincer grasp and could combine at the midline. She could stand and raise to a standing position, and she could walk with help and throw a ball. Object constancy had not moved beyond the 8–10 month level. There was, however, a more differentiated stranger reaction, although she had not progressed beyond the nine month level in overall objectal development.

At 18 months, A. was functioning approximately at the 15–16 month level of mental development and at the 14 month level of motor development. Her greatest gains were in performance on the mental scales. She could put nine cubes in a cup on command, and place beads in a box, and she could place all of the pegs in a pegboard in 42 seconds, the only member of its cohort to do so. She also closed a round box. She could stir the spoon and could build a two cube tower. She could show her shoes on request, and point to the parts of a doll at the 19 month level, her highest pass. Thus verbal expressive and receptive comprehension were developing.

The examiner at this age began to have an understanding of A.'s variable responsiveness during examinations. He noted a decline in her alertness and responsiveness midway in testing, in contrast to an initially bright and energetic manner. Previously, this apparent "fatiguing" was attributed to testing her during her usual naptime. Such was not the case this time, and we might speculate that A. particularly in view of her low birth weight might have a lower fatigue threshold. Perhaps this factor might account for some variability in her performance on the mental scales from one testing period to another. Six months ago A. clearly unwrapped the cube, but a similar response could not be elicited three months before. This time, A. did not dangle the ring as she clearly did three months ago."

At this age, A. could now walk by herself but did not walk sideways, nor backwards, nor stand on one foot with help. She could raise to a standing position from her side, her highest pass at the 21 month level and was the only member of its cohort to do so. However, she did not throw the ball as she had at the last testing.

Object constancy remained at the 8–10 month level, but as this test is given later in the examination, fatigue could have entered in. On the objectal scale, A. responded actively to mother's affective response, but showed no more marked response to mother's threatening than to her surprised face (12–15 months). However, she did clearly comply with mother's request and prohibition, scaled at the 15–17 month level. Constancy as to things lagged far behind constancy in relation to persons (person permanence), with affective development in between. The examiner noted: "It is interesting to note that while initially A. reacted with distress to brief separations from mother as did the other siblings, she seemed to be the only one who could be readily comforted by the examiners, and who allowed them to hold her in mother's absence with some degree of comfort."

It was decided to test the two birth weight children in this cohort at 21 months, although the others were not retested at this time. A. was functioning at approximately the 18–19 month level of mental development and at the 17 month level of motor development. A. made her greatest mental gains at this time. Her highest pass was in placing six blocks on the blue formboard (22.4 month level). She pointed to three pictures and identified all but one part of the doll. Recognition-receptive language appeared to be more advanced than expressive language. She was, however, beginning to use words to make wants known. She could find two objects, indicating ability to differentiate two objects hidden simultaneously in a series of single displacements. There continued to be some inconsistency in her performance on mental scales, and the range of items covered was broad. She missed some earlier and easier items, then successfully completing later and harder ones. The examiner felt in this session that fatigueability did not completely describe what was happening, and posited the possibility that negativism was entering in. "In contrast to dulling of alertness and responsiveness, A. vocally rejected items, saying unh-unh, and crying in frustration if pressed toward the end of the unusually long testing."

Motorically, A. now walked sideways but not backwards, stood with help on the right foot, and walked up the stairs. She did not throw the ball although reported by mother doing so at home.

There was considerable progress in object constancy. She searched for the invisibly placed safety pins (11–12 months) and passed three of the four trials required at the 18–20 month level in deducing the placement of the rabbit behind one of three screens. Although she did not pass the item, there was considerable movement toward this level.

Objectally, A. showed a more marked negative reaction to the threatening than to the surprised face, although she did not imitate mother's hand clapping (and imitative skills were not developed on the mental scale.) Affective responsiveness seemed to be clearly in the 12–15 month range, and more commensurate with the level of object constancy of things and persons. In this session, A. initiated contact with the examiner, releasing from mother/grandmother and walking to A., sitting down and engaging in a task, and interrupting to return to mother for "refueling". It also seemed that the unh-unh is a precursor to the third organizer, the No, suggestive of affective growth.

At 24 months, A. was functioning approximately at the 23 month level of mental development and at the 21 month level of motor development—clearing very cose to normative. Her mental development continued to accelerate. Her highest pass was in placing pegs in 22 seconds and in folding paper (both at 27 months). Her earliest failure was in naming one object (17–18 months). A.'s pattern was similar: she showed facility in fine motor manipulation of objects and form perception (pegs, six block tower, folding paper), but lagged behind in expressive language, although receptive and recognition language continued to develop well. She pointed correctly to five pictures and discriminated cup, box, plate on request (26 months). There continued to be some inconsistency of response, for example being unable to place six blocks of the blue formboard, which had been correctly done last time at 21 months. However, the waxing and waning of attention as well as the negativism seen previously was not in evidence.

Motorically, she now walked backwards, stood with help on both right and left feet, and walked up and down the stairs with help. She also could stand up from a side position; highest pass at 21.9 months.

On the object constancy scale, A. passed all trials in finding the rabbit behind three screens, at the 18–20 month level. (This is the highest criterion of the object constancy scale administered.)

Objectally, A. showed a delayed but clear reaction to the threatening face, at the 12–15 month level. Imitative skills have preceeded at a rapid pace (she could imitate folding a paper). She was able to work persistently and without distraction and with enjoyment even during mother's frequent absence during the session.

At age 30 months, the Stanford Binet, Form L-M intelligence test was given. No motor development test was administered. A. attained a mental age of 2-9, and IQ of 104 on the Binet, a 15 point increase over the Bayley MDI of 24 months. Basal was established at 2-0 and ceiling at 4-0. Her pattern of successes and failures was irregular. She did not pass the Picture Vocabulary test at II-6, passed only Picture Memory at III, but completed three tasks at the III-6 level (a sorting task and an interpretation of a picture's meaning, the only member of its cohort to do so; and a part-whole problem). Expressive language lagged somewhat behind receptive language, and A. seemed to know more than she was likely to show in words. Her ready comprehension of sorting instructions and her accurate interpretive comments suggest not only good memory and ability to maintain set, but also advance in reflective thinking.

Perceptual-motor skills did not seem as well developed, but were within average age limits. Four of six items of the 111 year level tap such skills, which may explain to some extent the unevenness of her performance.

Socially, A. was shy and subdued, but clearly alert and attentive. She was easily engaged in the "games" and generally persistent and attentive in problem solving. She also displayed admirable delay capacity, waiting for the next item's materials to be provided without fussing or distraction. She also took some initiative in "helping" the examiner replace used items in their proper boxes. Attention to task was somewhat interrupted by brief separations from mother who left the room several times. A. did not show distress, but verbalized desire to wait to play the games when mother returned.

At three, the examiner introduces his report with the following: "To my biased eyes, A. seems to be blossoming into a charming and bright little girl. She was indeed the most interpersonally engaging and responsive of the sibs." She did not show the fluctuation in energy and attention levels seen previously, suggesting more stamina and strength at this time. She also seemed to tolerate mother's absences from the room better than the other sibs. She also did not become low-keyed at these times nor verbalize that she wished to wait to reengage in the games.

Overall, A. received a Binet IQ of 131 with an MA of 4-2 and a CA of 3-0. Vocabulary and verbal conceptual ability stood out as relative areas of advance. She was credited at the 5-0 level with word definitions and pictorial similarities and differences. Her ceiling was at year VI and basal at III. There were two areas of relative weakness. She passed small muscle fine-motor coordination tasks at III, such as stringing beads, building a block bridge, copying a circle, and vertical line and sorting buttons at III-6. However, her movements were not smooth, but jerky, and she showed some overshoot and incoordination. Verbal expressive abilities were also less well developed, she did not pass response to pictures at III-6, giving only one-word replies. However, overall, there seemed to be a spurt in mental development, a positive acceleration rate reflected in testing since the 18 month period.

We can see from this progression that A. moved from developmental lag to above average mental performance. This child showed a mental spurt from 18 months and went on to develop a superior level of functioning by age 3. There was some variability of functioning with perceptual motor skills and expressive language not as well developed as other abilities. However, word definitions and vocabulary were at the 5 year level. There was a progression in motor development, but not to her chronological age, when tested at 24 months. This pattern is similar to the total group and cohort findings. It is my impression that the mental development scores reflect the influence of other than birthweight factors, such as socioeconomic status and parenting care, while the motor development scores reflect low birth weight and associated factors. It is also possible that there is a lower ceiling to the motor test.

As early as nine months, child A. began to discriminate mother from stranger, smiling only at the talking and silent mother. There was an early trend toward objectal development preceding object constancy. At 18 months, person permanence preceded affective development and object constancy lagged behind both. At this age also, she could be most readily of the other siblings be comforted by the examiners in mother's absence. This suggests a secure attachment to the mother from an early age, with the capacity to transfer this security to substitute persons.

Boy, B. I report at three months, that B. "in spite of his series of rehospitalizations, is functioning well." His mental functioning and motor functioning are within the second month of development. He passed two items in the fourth month on the motor scale. Sensory functioning was good, he did visually recognize the mother, but he did not as yet have a social discrimination. His head was balanced and he turned from back to side. At that time there was no object constancy reported, and he had reached the first criterion of the objectal scale (anticipation of feeding). During the examination, I noted that B. arched his back in what looked like a spastic movement.

At six months, B. was functioning at about the fourth month of mental development. He was visually regarding objects, and recognizing sounds, but not reaching out for objects or handling objects placed in his hands. He did exploit a piece of paper. Motorically, he could elevate himself by his arms, pull to a sitting position, and sit with slight support. His head was balanced, he turned from back to side, and he could hold his head steady. He also could turn from his back to his side. Object constancy was again not begun. He cooed at me, and smiled at mother when she was talking, suggesting an intermediary stage of objectal development. B. was last in developmental progress at this time, exceeding by A. who was lowest in birth weight, although he was last in birth order.

At nine months, B. was presently functioning at about the fifth month of mental development, and motor development as well. The major change since the last testing was that he was now grasping objects and he could carry them to his mouth. He could retain two cubes, and string, but not a pellet. There was some attention developed, such as attention to scribbling. He could sit momentarily, and roll from back to stomach. Object constancy had not developed. His level of object relations was undifferentiated, smiling at both examiner and mother. He could be quieted by the seen mother.

At a year of age, B. was functioning at about the eighth month level of mental development, and at the fifth month in motor development. He did gain three months in mental development since the last testing. The items contributing to this growth were such items as pulling the string to obtain the ring, lifting a cup by the handle, retaining two cubes offered to him, manipulating and ringing the bell, all requiring some motor response that might have been unavailable to him the previous testing. There was also some perceptual development. He looked for a fallen spoon, and found a hidden cube (suggesting some movement in object constancy). His response to the mirror suggested also some social development. There was some language precursor in his listening selectively to familiar words and saying "da-da" or its equivalent. He was also looking at pictures in a book.

Motor development was lagging. The only growth from the last testing was his ability to grasp a cube. He was not yet sitting alone, and the right hand was tightly closed, unless one placed something in it. During the objectal scale, it was noted again that he arched his back in somewhat spastic fashion.

B. was delayed as to object constancy, although he placed at the three to four month level on that scale. He was able to search for the dropped ball, but he could not reach for the invisible whole from a visible fraction, (six to nine months). Objectally, he showed no differentiation between examiner and mother, smiling and cooing at both. However, he did object to play with mother being interrupted, but not to the loss of an object. Thus, he had not moved beyond the five month level, that is negative effect at the loss of the human figure, but not at the point that displeasure is expressed at the loss of an object as well (nine months).

At this time I wrote: "Present results suggest more movement on the mental scale, with some delays in object constancy and objectal development. The motor delays and the delay in the use of the right hand, as well as the arching of the back, suggests that there might be some motor involvement. It was suggested that he be encouraged to use his right hand whenever possible to strengthen those muscles." We might note at the same time, however, that there had been movement in the mental scale on items requiring motor movements suggesting some improvements motorically since the last testing which showed up more on the mental than on the motor scale.

At 15 months, B. was functioning at the nine month level on the mental scale as compared with seven-eight month level three months previously. Motorically, he improved from the five-six month level to the nine-ten month level. The increments of development were as follows: He was now using his right hand more, and was able to transfer objects. He was vocalizing. He could cooperate in a game, and prehension had improved so that he attempted to grasp three cubes. He perceived the small hole in the pegboard and could finger it. He could find a hidden object, look for a hidden object, perceive pictures in a book, and in a social sense he could inhibit on command

and repeat a performance laughed at. There was some evidence that he was repeating words and using gestures to make his wants known. Motorically, there was considerable improvement He could sit alone for 30 seconds. There was complete thumb opposition in grasping a cube. There was ability to walk with help. He could sit down from a standing position. He also had midline skill in playing patti-cake.

In object constancy measures, B. was now at Criterion 3B (8-10 months) where he could find a stopwatch under a second screen. Objectally, he differentiated a stranger from mother, he could be comforted by the not-seen mother, at Criterion 3, and he was partially successful on Criterion 4 where he reacted positively to mother's playing with him but not negatively to an interruption or to removal of a toy. Objectally, he seemed to be at the fifth month, where he showed pleasure at frolic play with the mother, but he did not react negatively either to her loss or the loss of a toy. He was noted to imitate a sibling in manners, vocalization, and affective expression, which suggested better objectal development in relation to siblings than to mother. Also, B.'s response to mother's interruption of play and removal of a toy by the examiner was very similar to his reaction to the inhibition command, "No". He startled and became very alert and solemn. This suggests that he was more alert and aware and inhibited affective expression, and inhibition on command is at the tenth month of development.

I noted: "B. seems to have made impressive development, having gained four months motorically in three months. It appears that this is his present spurt, with also evidence of a fair amount of social and mental awareness that was not present before" or we might add, expressed overtly. There is some suggestion that there was more awareness than had been capable of being expressed earlier.

At 18 months, B. was presently functioning at the fourteenth month of mental development, as compared with 11 months at the three months previous testing. His highest successes were placing a circle in the Blue Board at 14 months, and saying two words at 14 months. There was a very hesitant, quiet and shy manner of relating from this infant and considerable sensitivity. I noted that it took longer for him to engage than his brother, and that he objected to loud sounds. However, if I made less noise and a game out of the quieter sounds, he showed interest and evident enjoyment. There was also a need to mouth objects before he engaged actively with them, as if he had to engage in soothing behavior to become organized. At present, he engaged in adaptive memory functioning, looked at pictures, imitated a scribble, remembered and unwrapped a cube, uncovered a box, turned the pages of a book, and engaged in other imitative behavior. His fine motor coordination was quite good, even though I reported that he continued to favor the left hand and the right hand was now completely relaxed. There was reported some awkwardness in two-handed tasks. There was evident progress in the verbal area.

Motor functioning was at the tenth month, with highest success on throwing a ball at the thirteenth month. While he was presently walking with help, he was not standing alone or walking by himself. New items of functioning were being able to combine objects at the midline and sitting alone with good coordination. "It is in this area that he is most behind the other infants. It is possible that if strength for locomotion does not increase, some physiotherapy might be beneficial".

On the object constancy scale, B. was at the base of locating a doubly displaced object under one screen but not under two screens, between the eighth and tenth month of object constancy, no movement since last testing. On the other hand, he had moved dramatically on the objectal scale. Here he was reported to kiss mother: he could respond to a request and to a prohibition (15-17 month level), and he responded positively to mother's play (12th month level) and affectively to mother's negative affect (12-15 months). These findings demonstrated considerable emotional and social awareness and sensitivity. "It was as if he has had to concentrate in this area because of the other delays, and this both was an aid and a hindrance". "It made him more responsive to the frustration of his limitations. Hence, behaviorally, he must be handled with an eye to the sensitivities and frustrations he is experiencing. We would recommend that he be removed when he is over-stimulated and overly frustrated rather than punished, and that the biting behavior (reported by parents) be handled in the same manner".

Both low birth weight children were seen at the hospital at 21 months for an interim checkup although the cohort was now going to be seen every six months. B. arrived very unhappy and had to be rolled around in his stroller before he could be quieted. A. was tested first as she seemed in a happy frame of mind. As she was achieving a growth spurt, her testing took quite a length of time. While B. had quieted down, and he had had his lunch, it was obvious to me that he was quite fatigued. As a result, I tested him quite quickly, and asked his grandmother to hold him on her lap for the testing and he seemed happy and comfortable with her. I feared he would again start crying if placed in the baby chair.

Even though he was quite fatigued, he did somewhat better on this testing than on the previous testing. The developmental items that he added were: pushing car along; putting cubes in a cup; imitating patting of the whistle doll; imitation of words; putting beads in a box; building a tower of two cubes; saying two words, by report; using gestures to make wants known; showing shoe; and placing pegs in a pegboard in 70 seconds. His highest passes were at 17.0 and 17.6 months, where he attained a toy with a stick, and named one object. These items were both verbal and nonverbal. There seemed to be development of imitative behavior as a precursor to speech, and some evident efforts at speech.

Motor coordination had improved. The items that were added had to do with increasing motor coordination. He could now stand alone, and pull himself to a standing position, and stand on his right foot with help. He pulled himself up on furniture very well. In addition, he was capable of using his right hand with increasing skill, and reached with this hand and held a cookie with it.

On the object constancy scale, B. was now able to function at item 4A, where he could find the safety pins under one screen but not under two (11-12 months). On the objectal scale, he responded with a delayed reaction to mother's threatening face, similar to his response of three months ago. He was also the baby who was most frightened by the new situation of the hospital, suggesting that he retained some stranger anxiety. He was described last time as being the most sensitive of the babies. The conclusion at this time was that he was more than holding his own and was making some improvements. Considering this fatigue, we felt that these test results were minimal and further testing would be done in the family home.

At home, on his second birthday, B. was again crying and irritable. When the examiner presented him with cubes, however, he suddenly became interested in the testing, and responses after this were quick, and punctuated by his insistent request for more. At this time, there was an evident growth spurt on the mental scale. The MDI became normative, 81 for birth age. His best successes were with some nonverbal items (putting pegs in a pegboard, mending a broken doll, differentiating scribble from stroke), but there was also evident receptive language and some expressive language. This was a dramatic spurt from the birth age MDI of 58 three months ago. At present, he was functioning more like a 20 month infant.

While the spurt was not as dramatic on the motor scale, there was also an increase in PDI. He had taken several steps and was on the point of walking. While he did not use his right hand for most things, there was more use of the right hand than previously noted. He was walking upstairs and downstairs on his hands and knees, and he could raise himself from a supine position.

Objectally, he reached the 12–15 month level on the scale, of differentiating the astonished from the prohibiting mother. On the object constancy scale, he had reached the 18–20 month level where he could find the object under three screens, quite an advance over the previous testing. This is the highest criterion level for that scale.

At two and a half, B. was given the Stanford Binet Form L-M Intelligence test. He attained a mental age of 2-5 and IQ of 94 which compared with an MDI of 91 for gestation age six months ago, and 81 for birth age. He was now clearly functioning in the average range of intelligence. His best performance was on pictorial memory, but he also did well with verbal and verbal memory items. He tended to have difficulty with motor items, and where possible these were omitted from the scoring (using alternate items). It was noted that he was still more comfortable using his left hand, but he was using his right hand more.

He was quite fitful in the beginning of the testing, and somewhat withholding. He found it difficult to separate from mother. He was being toilet trained and we wondered whether the negativism was related to this, We might also note that this might be considered to represent the third organizer, and in this sense, an emotional advance.

B. was again tested with the Binet at three years. He attained a mental age of 3-3 and IQ of 104. He obtained a basal at age 11, five months credit at age II-6, two months credit at age III, three months credit at age III-6, two months credit at age IV, two months credit at age IV-6, one month credit at age V, and a ceiling at age VI. This is a very wide spread and range of testing, most unusual even at this age. His earlier failure was on Identifying Objects by Use at II-6, but subsequently the major difficulties have to do with nonverbal, motor items such as failing Stringing Beads at age III and Sorting Buttons at III-6. His motor problem was in evidence, and he became frustrated easily. His best functioning was on verbal items, passing Definitions at age V, Comprehension and Three Commissions at IV-6, and Opposite Analogies and Discrimination of Forms, where motor involvement is not necessary, at age IV.

What was noted during this testing is that when he is feeling unable to do tasks, his involvement is minimal, and he complained that he was not feeling well. It was noted that he still favored the left hand, and had difficulty in coordination when there was a two-handed task. "Clearly verbal functioning was his forte, and he knew three vocabulary words for the VI year level".

The conclusion was that the wide spread and superior verbal functioning suggested that this result was only an estimate, possibly an underestimate, and that future tests with scales with less motor materials might rate him higher.

B. showed a consistent pattern of motor development delay. This difficulty in motor development was noted in testing, when he was seen to have a problem with tasks requiring the use of his right hand. He was also late in motor development milestones such as sitting and walking. This is consistent with the findings of research on children with medical complications (Piper, Mazer, Silver, & Ramsay, 1988; Landry, Chapieski, Fletcher, & Denson, 1988.) However, by the age of two and a half, B. had attained average mental status. His major difficulties continued to be with motor items, but verbal abilities were superior by age three.

Objectal development preceded object constancy in the early months, but both were delayed as were mental and motor development. At fifteen months, while object constancy was at the 8–10 month level, the measured objectal score was at five months. However, clinical observations noted inhibition of command at the tenth month and a social response and imitation of siblings. There was a dramatic shift in both mental score and on the objectal scale at 18 months. This was accompanied by an observation of emotional awareness and sensitivity that was manifested in overt negativism and response to frustration in both the testing situation and at home. We are beginning to see a pattern of relationship between objectal functioning and mental functioning which is most dramatic in this infant because of his motor delay. Also, while the motor functioning was relatively delayed in this child at age three, verbal functioning was at a superior level.

Middle Birth Weight Examples

Girl, A. The two children to be described below represent an intermediate birth weight of our cohorts, but were of shorter gestation than the quintuplets, who were smaller for date.

At three months, A. was described to us as being very cranky this week, not being content even when being held. She was also described as having been the good baby who never cried until this time. Her sleep schedule was different from the others in the cohort.

Present test functioning was at the 2.6 month level. Her responses were described as definite and crisp. She smiled on hearing sounds, and her best functioning to mental items was her capacity to localize the source of sound from two objects and to transfer her attention back and forth between the two objects. Good attention, and sensitivity as well as emerging development of object constancy was suggested.

The motor functioning was at the 3.7 level of development, with one item at the fourth month. She could elevate herself prone, could sit propped on mother's lap, and had an initial grasp, and could balance her head for short periods of time.

Although there were indications of emerging object constancy, she did not succeed on the Décarie at the third to fourth month. On the objectal scale, she did pass Criterion 1, the feeding response. For Criterion 2, she smiled at both the silent and talking mother, and at the examiner, although she did not coo at the examiner. It was noted that when fed and napped, she did well in the testing situation and was happy and contented. Mother noted a shorter attention span than the others, and a recommendation was made that her schedule be altered to fit her own pattern of behavior.

At six months, A. was an attractive petite baby, very alert and interested in her environment. Her successes ranged from the 4th month to the 5.8 month. Growth was approximately two and a half months in a three month period. She was aware of a strange situation, inspected her own hands, attended to sounds in the environment. She looked intently at her own image in the mirror and discriminated strangers. She turned her head at a vanishing spoon. She was able to actively manipulate the table, exploit paper and string, and bang in play, using primarily her right hand. However, she was not yet actively grasping objects. She vocalized attitudes, but had a small range of sound production.

The range of motor functioning was from 4.2 months to 5.7 months (rotating the wrist). Additional items at this time were sitting with slight support, pulling to a sitting position, sitting momentarily, and unilateral reaching. Sitting and prehension was slower to develop.

Object constancy had not yet been reached, and A. was described as having very little interest in objects. Affectively, she scored at about the fifth month of development. She smiled at the examiner and the silent and talking mother. She could be quieted by the seen and the absent mother, at the fifth month. In the home, she demanded constant attention from mother. She seemed to be overstimulated by the sight and activity of others, but quieted down when placed in her own room. It was our impression that there might be some delay in CNS development and hyperalertness to external and internal stimuli, requiring more naps and some removal from overstimulation. We earlier found that frequent naps and small feedings were of help to her. She additionally also seemed to get most of her sense of well being from optimal contacts with mother.

A. was quiet, shy, reserved, and slow to get into the testing situation at nine months, but once in was quite capable and responsive. Functioning on the mental scale was close to 8.9 months. The items that were added had to do with prehension (capacity to secure cubes, to manipulate string and bell), verbal receptive items such as listening selectively to familiar words, saying da-da, and evidences of maturing object constancy, such as cooperating in peekaboo games, uncovering a toy, and inhibiting on command. On the motor scale, functioning was close to 8.1 months. The items that were added were improved prehension for cube and pellet, sitting alone with good coordination, stepping progression, standing by furniture, and raising self to standing and sitting position.

In object constancy, functioning was at the 8–10 month level. She was able to follow a fallen ball, discriminate a pencil from a fraction, but she also was able to find the vanished object under two screens. On the objectal scale, she was pleased with mother's attention, but as with the other infants, showed her displeasure at her loss only with a change in facial expression. The infants in this cohort seemed to be able to tolerate the absence of mother without visible upset. This item scores at the fifth month. The nine month test, negative reaction to loss of toy is also not expressed vocally, although her facial expression did change.

At one year, A. was pleasant, sweet, and engaging. Mental functioning was at nine months of age, and there was a relatively restricted range of functioning. The items that were added were vocalizing four different syllables, picking up and securing a cube, responding to a verbal request, and inhibiting on command. On the motor scale, she added items having to do with combining spoons in the midline, stepping movements, fine prehension of the pellet, and patticake.

On the object constancy scale, A. was able to find the stopwatch, one visible displacement, but she did not make use of a sequence of invisible displacements. Object constancy was between 8 and 10 months. She was at the ninth month of development on the objectal scale, but more definitely responded negatively to the interruption of mother's playing and negatively to the loss of a toy. We felt at this time that the relative slow rate of development since the last testing related to a sharp jump in the scale at this age level.

A. showed a spurt in mental functioning at 15 months. Her best functioning was on items having to do with language and gesture at the 15th month level (shows dress, uses gestures to make wants known, says two words). She was also skillfull on items requiring prehension and grasping, as well as imitation (places round blocks, removes pellet from bottle, patting whistle doll in imitation, to the 14th month level). It was interesting to note that mother introduced her as the smartest.

However, on the motor side of functioning, she was not yet walking. She was standing and walking with help, but continued to prefer to crawl. She had midline skills and could play patticake. Objectally, she reached Criterion 6 at the 15–17 month level, that is she could comply with both a request and a prohibition. On Criterion 7, she imitated mother's hand clapping but did not respond affectively to mother's threatening face. On the object constancy scale, she could find two safety pins under one screen, and one safety pin under two screens, at the 11–12 month level.

A. was viewed as small and petite, very quick to relate to the examiner, and just as quick in all her responses at her 18 month birthday. Running throughout this testing session was her difficulty in taking risks, pushing things to the examiner to do for her. Thus, there was some loss of score on the mental tests. She did add the following items: turning pages of the book; dangling ring by the string; putting beads in a box; placing one peg repeatedly; building a tower of two cubes; spontaneous scribble; putting nine crubes in a cup; closing round box; building a tower of three cubes; and attaining a toy with a stick. Her use of language was unstable, although she did not speak two words to the examiner. Some tests, such as putting the round block in last time, she failed to do this time. It was felt that her refusal to do something difficult for herself accounted for the variability of functioning.

A. was not yet walking, and it was felt this related to her difficulty of taking risks. She did stand alone, stood up from first and second levels, and could stand on right and left feet with help.

Objectally, she showed a more negative reaction to mother's threatening than to her surprised face; and had already responded to both a request and a prohibition. She did not pass the object constancy scale at the 18–20 month level. She was able to find the safety pins under one screen, but when a second screen was added she reached for the box rather than looking for the pins where they were. Object constancy appeared to be at the 11–12 month level. This delay in object constancy was felt to be related to and account for the inability to risk and make an attempt to solve difficult problems. If she could not retain the object in memory, it might be difficult to solve such things as the Blue Board.

A. at two years was shy and slow to warm up to the examiner, and murmured in a sweet quiet voice. While still shy and tentative, she was more willing to take risks and was less needing of mother to do things for her. She was spontaneous and smiling at the examiner and particularly enjoyed the motor scale. She later imitated the examiner by wearing glasses.

She was able to respond to three of the Picture Vocabulary items of the Stanford Binet, Form L-M Intelligence test, so this scale was administered rather than the Bayley. She achieved a mental age of 2-4 and an IQ of 114. This represented a real growth spurt since the Bayley at 18 months. Her most solid functioning was at year 11, where she passed all items, both verbal and nonverbal. At year II-6 she could identify objects by use, parts of the body, and perform the Three-Hole formboard rotated. She was less able to pass verbal items as their level of difficulty increased. At III, she was able to draw a vertical line, and failed all items at the III-6 level.

At two years, she could now walk up and down stairs with help, stand up with little assistance, and could stand on each foot alone. She did not jump or walk backwards. She achieved object constancy at 18–20 months, thus having caught up to the objectal level of the scale.

A. was shy during the two and one half year old testing. She refused the Picture Vocabulary test initially, but later was able to do it. She refused repetition of digits. She tended at times to fade out but generally was cooperative and interested in the test items. She clearly was interested in the adults, and remained with us after testing was completed. She was reluctant to have the testing end.

She attained a mental age of 3-1 and resultant IQ of 117, on the Binet at age two and a half. Her highest successes were on perceptual discrimination items: Discrimination of Forms at year IV, and Pictorial Similarities and Differences at year IV-6 (the latter often seen as a screening item for reading readiness). She also passed Response to Pictures at year III-6, suggesting well developed verbal abilities. Some of her early failures in this testing seemed to relate to overall inhibition. It was felt that the measure was probably an underestimate of her intellectual abilities at that time.

A. continued to be her shy self, warming up the examiner only gradually, at three years of age. She spoke softly, and had to be encouraged, but finally began to enjoy the testing, so much so that she did not want to leave the room at the end of the session. She was also clearly doing well, obtaining a mental age of 3-11 at three years of age, and a resultant IQ of 123 on the Binet.

Her best functioning was in the verbal area, with Definitions passed at the V year level. She was also advanced in nonverbal areas. Highest passes were on Aesthetic Comparison and Pictorial Similarities and Differences at year IV-6. All functioning was clearly above her chronological level. She also had a very definite idea of herself as the "sister" in the family, giving this as one of her responses.

This child represents a middle birthweight child, with the lowest birth weight in her cohort. She showed the similar pattern of verbal spurt ending in above average intelligence, and motoric delay (not walking at eighteen months). There was some early delay in both mental and motor functioning, and hyperalertness and response to overstimulation noted at 6 months. She demonstrated a mental spurt at 15 months. This spurt, as in the previous infant, was accompanied by a spurt in objectal score. By age 2, she was functioning at the bright normal level of intelligence, and by age 3 all functioning was above her chronological level with best functioning in the verbal area.

Boy, B. B. was a very sturdy baby, described at three months as being strong and tough to the touch. He did well on both mental and motor scales of the Bayley. On the mental scale, he was functioning at about the second month of development with the following items passed: anticipatory adjustment to lifting, 2.6; fingers hands in play, 3.2; and inspecting hands, 3.8. He vocalized two different sounds, reacted to the disappearance of a face, searched for sound, and vocalized to E's social smile and talk.

On the motor scale, his functioning was at about the fourth month. His head was well balanced, he sat with slight support, and could grasp a cube, ulnar-palmar prehension. His hands were predominantly open, he elevated himself by his arms prone, and could turn from side to back.

He had not yet achieved object constancy. He could not follow a disappearing ball. Objectally, he reacted to the feeding situation by sucking and turning to mother. He smiled at the examiner during the testing situation but not on the Décarie Scale. He did smile at the talking mother. He did not differentiate between mother and stranger.

At six months of age, B. was functioning at the five and one half month level of mental development and at approximately birth age, six months, in motor development. His highest pass was in making a playful response to the mirror (the only quad to do so), and his earliest failure was in retaining two cubes. He secured one cube and the pellet. He also transferred objects from hand to hand. His reaching, however, was not deft and direct. Interest in vocal sound productions was emerging. He was reported to have vocalized three syllables. He also attended to scribbling.

On the motor scale, B. passed items between 5.7 and 6.8 months, (scooping the pellet). He could sit momentarily for 15 seconds alone. He rotated his wrist, had partial thumb opposition, and turned from back to side but not from back to stomach.

Object constancy lagged behind objectal development; he did not follow the disappearing ball where it fell, but he turned his head to accommodate visually to a rolling but not disappearing ball. Objectally, he cooed and smiled at the silent examiner, and smiled at both the smiling and talking mother. He responded positively to the seen and unseen-talking mother, and reacted positively to her play. He did not yet react negatively to its interruption. Objectal development appeared to be solidly on the five month level.

At nine months, B. was found to have shown a radical shift in behavior as well as functioning on the tests. He was described as remaining socially sensitive, that is he could inhibit to command at the 10 month level, and continued to have a playful response to the mirror. However, mother described a recent mood shift, in that he seemed more lethargic, unhappy and unresponsive, much like a depressed baby. During the testing, he maintained a vacant, glassy stare, with only marginal interest and attention to task or situation, mouthed and sucked objects, drooled and engaged in cranky crying toward the end of the test. He was being tested during naptime, however, at the same age the other quads also were and were more alert. Mother presented a picture of a situation in which she has tended to leave the quads much to themselves to deal with their competition for her attention. B. was the last to be picked up because he was the one who was so good i.e. he made less insistent and overt demands on her attention, in contrast to a brother who screamed. It was felt that he might be more sensitive to being left alone, and yet less able to make his needs known.

As a result of this emotional slump, B. functioned at a decline at the seven to eight month level on both the mental and motor tests at nine months. He could not retain a second cube, 4.7 months, and did not reach for the third cube. He did not hold objects simultaneously in each hand. Grasping was tentative and awkward. Frequently, he would close on an object and after initial contact immediately release it, as if dropping a hot potato. It was noted by his examiner that a fine motor delay was possible, and should be charted in later testings. B. also did not seem alert to detail nor very interested in manipulating objects. He did not manipulate the bell although he did ring it. He did not pick up the cup nor look for contents of the box. He was not saying four syllables, but he was listening selectively and could say da-da.

On the motor scale, his range of items passed was between 6.7 months and 8.6 months, with an uneven pattern. He had prewalking progression, crawling on all fours, but did not have stepping movements. He pulled to standing and could stand by furniture, but he could not raise himself to a sitting position nor lower himself from standing to sitting. There was not complete thumb opposition, and he did not combine at the midline. Transfer across the midline was noted but awkward.

Object constancy was between six and nine months. B. followed the ball and attempted to grasp the reappearing partial pencil. He did not actively search for a vanished object. Objectally, B. showed a minimal pleasure response to play with mother. He seemed alert to her, and quieted his crying and briefly smiled, but he did not vocalize his pleasure. He showed a negative nonverbal reaction to interruption of his play. Some suggestions were made concerning more attention being paid to B., e.g. picking him up sooner than later. There was an additional note at this time, also, that he may have reacted more to an illness on vacation and separation from mother during a parental vacation. With the recommendation concerning more attention, B. was back to his smiley self in a week".

There was a discrepancy in mental and motor functioning at one year, possibly partially related to what may be a sharp jump in the mental scale. B. made some advance in motor development, to the nine to ten month level, but mental functioning remained at the eight month level overall, similar to the last testing.

The decrease in the mental scale was somewhat deceptive as the decrease was accounted for by B.'s continued lag in manipulation of objects (grasping, reaching, securing, exploring detail). He still did not retain two of three cubes, nor attempt to secure the third cube. He did not manipulate the bell. Grasping continued to be one-sided and not bilateral. Midline behavior was absent and there continued to be difficulty of inhibition to release, i.e. dropping objects like a hot potato on contact. His contact with objects was banging. He listened selectively, vocalized, said da-da, and inhibited on verbal command. He had a neat pincer, and fingered the holes in a pegboard. He seemed more interested in distal than close visual stimuli; for example, observing a bird in the tree outside the window through a series of position moves. Yet he had difficulty manipulating near objects, and he was the only quad to focus on and "look" at pictures in a book.

It was wondered whether his lag in manipulation of objects might relate to a spurt in gross motor areas, specifically in walking. He was the only quad to walk with help at this age, and his stepping movements were quite vigorous. However, use of both body sides and midline activity continued to be absent, with right side preferred. There was some concern at this testing whether the lag in manipulation of objects signalled a minimal cerebral dysfunction.

Objectally, B. did not imitate mother's affectionate response, consistent with lack of imitation on mental scale items. On the object constancy scale, he did actively search and secure the safety pins through a single, invisible displacement, the only quad to do so, at the 10–11 month level. Affectively, B. was highly attentive and expressive in person contact, with the depressive manner seen in the previous testing not evident.

At 15 months, there was a growth spurt in both mental and motor development. Language development in the mental area continued to be an area of advance. Highest passes were in using gestures (14.6 months), and saying two words (14.2). Lag was still evident in the manipulation of objects. In this testing, it was less related to lack of ability to release, and more to distinct preference to secure and hold onto objects. His earliest failure was in putting a cube in a cup on command. B. seemed more interested in securing the cube placed in the cup by the examiner. He was more interested in detail at this time, and rang the bell purposively. He showed curiosity in manipulating objects. Grasping had become bilateral. However, while he secured two cubes, they were not integrated at the midline and he did not play patticake or bang spoons or cubes in imitation. He mouthed objects but was teething. He could place one round block in the form board, and fingered the peg board repeatedly, but he did not place a peg, or place objects in containers.

Motorically, his gross motor skills showed advance, relative also to his sibs. B. walked sideways and backwards, threw a ball, and stood and walked alone. Gross motor skills were advanced over fine motor skills.

Objectally, B. still did not imitate mother's affectionate response, although some imitative ability was demonstrated on the mental scale, such as rolling a car. It was wondered whether he could not blow a kiss as the other quads did because of the delay in development of midline skill. He showed some progress objectally beyond the 11 month level, in other areas. He complied with a request but not a prohibition, and had a more marked reaction to threatening than to a surprised face, but without gestural imitation of hand clapping, again a midline activity.

As to object constancy, he made active search for a vanished object with a sequence of invisible displacements at the 11–12 month level. He passed two of five items at the 18–20 month level, suggesting that this was emerging. For B. the décalage or discrepancy between objectal development and object constancy seemed to be in favor of objects, in contrast to his siblings, where objectal development preceded. This seems inconsistent with his difficulties in manipulation of objects. However, it was noted by his examiner that he had an interest in objects, often distal ones, and it may be that his very frustration and difficulty at manipulation contributed to his attention to and cathexis of objects and his greater advance in this area. A contributing factor also to the décalage may have been his difficulty in asserting his wants in competition with more verbally outspoken siblings, resulting for a brief time in less attention.

Some environmental and experimental changes occurred at the 18 month testing. Mother described B. as being more attached to mother at this time, in contrast to a previous ability to go to strangers. This change occurred since they lost a day girl to whom he was attached two months previously, and also since parental vacation. We wondered whether he had not experienced some separation anxiety at these events. Mother was feeling stressed because of the demands of four infants at once with his added clinging. Another change at this time was that of examiner.

There was little change in the rate of functioning mentally since the last testing, but with language development not as well developed as nonverbal skills. Items added were: Putting three more cubes in a cup; turning the pages of a book, patting the whistle doll; putting beads in a box; placing one peg; removing the pellet from a bottle; building a tower of two cubes; spontaneous scribble; putting nine cubes in a cup; closing the round box; round block in pink board; and attaining a toy with stick. These items indicate motoric advancement and growth in imitative skills. Motor development was relatively improved over the last testing. The items added were: standing on one foot, walking upstairs with help; and getting upright from a supine position.

At this time, he had achieved beyond the last criterion of the objectal scale, as suggested by his increased interest and rapprochement crisis with his mother. Object constancy was at the 18–20 month level, at age or above. It would seem that the décalage previously noted had been bridged. He demonstrated increased person relatedness. It was noted at this testing that all four infants needed more verbal contact and encouragement. The lack of gain in mental tests seemed to be related to the delay in language. All had minimal words achieved, with limited ability in one infant to point to three pictures.

B. was tested at two years by his original examiner. He was quiet, pleasant and sociable, and took the initiative in engaging his examiner. However, he also became shy, teary, and turned away and clung to mother when tests were introduced. His examiner engaged him with the Picture Vocabulary book, which he hung onto as testing proper was started, much as a transitional object. It was noted that he responded to new situations irritably and needed more time to do so with some opportunity for active participation in transitions.

B. made big gains in mental functioning since the last testing (although as noted above, previous test results might not have been optimal because of separations and change of examiner at that time). He attained a mental age of 2-5 and IQ of 118 on the Stanford Binet, Form L-M Intelligence test. Basal was at II and ceiling at III, with five subtests passed at the II-6 level. Identifying objects by name, the alternate at the II year level, was given as he balked at the delayed search for a hidden object, although his object constancy functioning was adequate for this task. Language functions tapped at this level were seen as adequately developing (identifying objects by name and pictorial representation). Short term memory (repeating two digits) was age appropriate, and he passed the form board. Although he did not pass stringing beads at III, he did seem to understand the task, in stringing one bead which he removed. The tasks failed at II-6 were obeying simple commands and Picture Vocabulary.

Motor development was age adequate. B. could stand on either foot alone and jumped off the floor with both feet. He could not walk up and down the stairs with help nor jump from the bottom step. Objectal and object constancy scales were both at criterion. B. seemed to have difficulty with tasks that necessitated letting go, which was felt might relate to timing for toilet training and need for care in transitions that would induce separation anxiety. Another thought about this is the long period of time in his learning to manipulate objects when he had difficulty with just this task, obtaining objects and then suddenly dropping them like a hot potato; followed by needing to cling to objects.

At two and a half years, B. is described as having a winning smile, used perhaps somewhat indiscriminately. His seeming social ability was felt not to be as socially understanding as his smile suggested. There was observed some mild impulsiveness, wanting to plunge ahead into a task without waiting for instructions. This gave the appearance at times of willfulness. He seemed alert, and showed something akin to humour, playing a joke with balkiness. On one occasion, it seemed a combination of impulsiveness, winning smile, and willingness to go along with the examiner, and turning it into a joke.

B. received a mental age of 3-0 and IQ of 115 on the Stanford Binet, Form L-M Intelligence test at two and a half. Basal was at II-6 and ceiling at IV-0. B. passed four tests at the III year level and two at the III-6 level. B.'s highest pass was Response to Pictures at III-6 where he gave two or more details for all three pictures. Picture Vocabulary was his earliest failure at III-0. Motor items, copying, stringing beads were marginally passed at III-0, with some awkwardness and overshooting more in evidence than with his sibs. It was felt that his motor development continued to be an area in which close tracking should be done.

At three years of age, B. was the last quad tested and his examiner was concerned about fatigue effects altering his performance. He was the only one asking to stop the testing, although he could be drawn back with relative ease. There was some suggestion that B.'s requests to stop playing the games might have had something to do with item difficulty or frustration on difficult items. B. tended to handle difficulties otherwise by quick comments that he "forgot", covered by a pleasing smile. His concentration on task and on doing task tended to be shorter than for the other quads, either in persisting in the face of difficulty or in delaying while instructions were completed. He plunged ahead on sorting buttons, and this task had to be repeated several times.

B. received a mental age of 3-8 and IQ of 116 on the Stanford Binet, From L-M Intelligence test, at age three. Basal was at III-0 and ceiling at year VI. B. passed four items at the III-6 level, two at IV, and one each at the IV-6 and V year levels. B.'s best functioning was on visual-perceptual tasks, such as Form Discrimination at IV, Patience Pictures, III-6, and Patience Rectangles at V. B. displayed concentration in problem solving with some pleasure in repeating the task. The only other task completed successfully beyond the IV year level was Pictorial Similarities and Differences at year IV-6.

His examiner wondered whether conceptual development in nonverbal modes outstripped verbal conceptual and expressive development. Comprehension and Vocabulary items at all levels tested beyond III tended to be poorly done and to elicit the requests to stop the testing most frequently. He was also below the other sibs in test results, which conflicted with mother's statements which seemed to go out of the way to present B. as advanced over the other sibs. At that time, we speculated that mother may have been having some uneasiness at B.'s progress.

His examiner felt that impressionistically, there was something dysfunctional in his performance, such as the overshooting on button sorting, as well as the verbal and word finding difficulties, impulsiveness, and confabulative tendencies. I quote: "One wonders if the visual-perceptual advance shown in part-whole tasks might be a splinter skill, or might reflect heightening of body image advance that might make B. in one sense sensitive to disparities in ability levels between self and sibs that might enforce passive, ingratiating, perhaps mirroring tendencies in coping style".

Quad B is a middle birthweight child who showed subtle problems with fine motor coordination noted from the age of 9 months: difficulty with midline tasks and with prehension, that is, dropping objects like "hot potatoes" and later difficulty in letting go of objects. Gross motor coordination in contrast was advanced over the other quads. This was accompanied by sensitivity to fatigue and separations, such as parental vacations, and a subsequent rapprochement crisis with mother resulting in clinging to mother at 18 months. By age 2 he had achieved the bright normal level of intelligence, but with a pattern of better performance on perceptual than verbal materials.

This quad showed dissimilarity in pattern from the infants previously described. At 15 months there was a mental and motor spurt, with continued difficulty in the manipulation of objects, and accompanying this there was a décalage with object constancy outstripping the objectal level. He seemed to favor objects and to pay attention to distal events (observing a bird outside the window). By 18 months the décalage had disappeared, but what remained in his pattern of testing was a clear relative strength on visual-perceptual tasks with relative difficulty on such verbal tasks as comprehension and vocabulary.

High Birth Weight Examples

Girl C. When C. was seen at three months, she was functioning above the three month level on both mental and motor tests. Her highest pass on the mental scale was approaching the mirror (4.4 months); and her earliest failure on this scale was visually tracking the ball at 3.1 months. Motorically, the head was steady and well balanced (4.2 months). Hands were not predominantly open and she was not reaching and grasping. Objectally, she reached Criterion 3, quieting with the seen and heard mother, at three months, but was not quieted by the heard and unseen mother. She did not track the rolling ball at Criterion I of the object constancy scale.

C. was seen by a new examiner at six months, because of the departure of her previous examiner. She was described as a "healthy, pleasant, contemplative looking infant who gazed fixedly at the stranger . . .". Her tension was expressed with a startle reaction when the examiner accidently banged a metal object against the table. She seemed shyer than the other siblings and was a bit slower to move into the testing, but was cooperative.

She passed all the mental tests through 6.3 months. Her first failure was "manipulating the bell with interest in detail", at 6.5 months. She then passed some items at the seven month level, including pulling a string to secure a toy, ringing a bell purposively, and saying da-da. Motor functioning was also at the six month level. She could sit alone for 30 seconds (6.0 level), but did not roll from back to stomach (6.4).

On the objectal scale, C. scored at Criterion 4 (5th month level), smiling at her mother during play and reacting with displeasure at having the play interrupted. Object constancy had moved to the six to nine month level, as she could reach for the fraction of the invisible whole object. (pencil).

C. was tested at nine months again by a different examiner. Her shyness resulted in a number of refusals which interfered with best functioning on the mental scale. Her highest success was on jabbering expressively at the 12.0 month level, her lowest failure was on retaining two cubes at the 6.2 level, more a function of her shyness. She did very well on the motor scale, with highest pass on midline skill at 9.7 months, and sitting down at 9.2 months. She was also standing by furniture at this time. She passed Criterion 4 on the objectal scale, reacting pleasurably to mother's play and negatively to interruption of that play and negatively to the loss of a toy, at the nine month level. Her ability to pass 4A and 4B of the object constancy scale (finding the object under two screens) suggested better intellectual functioning than her shyness permitted her to demonstrate on the mental scale.

C. continued her shy behavior during the 12 month testing, but the delay in initiating the examination was less than during the previous testing. Her highest successes were evenly divided between verbal and nonverbal items on the mental scale. Her highest scores were on using gestures to make wants known, closing a round box, putting nine cubes in a cup, and saying two words, all at the 14 month level. Her lowest failure was in holding a crayon adaptively, with no opportunity for this reported at home. She functioned between the 11 to 13 month level on the motor scale. She threw a ball, could stand alone briefly, had midline skill, and could pull herself down to a sitting position. Objectally, she was at the 15-17 month level, on Criterion 6, responding to both a request and a prohibition. She continued to have superior functioning on the object constancy scale. She passed at the highest criterion, 18-20 month level, finding the hidden object under three screens.

C. continued to have stranger anxiety at the beginning of the 15 month testing, but could gradually be introduced into the testing. She was able to whisper verbal responses in spite of her shyness, and her functioning became easier and freer as the examination progressed. Her functioning on mental tests was at the superior level. Her highest scores were in two word sentences (hi daddy) and naming two objects, ball and cup, at 20-6 months. Other high successes were on Naming one picture (cup) at 19.3 months, pointing to parts of the doll at 19.1 months, using words to make wants known and following directions on the doll at 17.8 months. C was now saying the following words: all gone, bye bye, dada, mama, hi, teeth, up, down, eye, fine, cook cook, poo poo, ow, no, yu, yum, show, sh sh baby, spoon, ball, doll, and teetee for TV. Her motor development was between the 12 and 16 month level. She was now walking, able to throw a ball, stand up from a supine position by rolling onto her stomach, walk sideways and backwards, and stand on each foot alone with help. Objectal and object constancy scales were both passed at the highest criterions (15-17 month and 18-20 month levels).

C. was more outgoing and less frightened by the examiner during the 18 month testing. There was some distractibility during the testing on naming and pointing to pictures, and mother was concerned that these tests be repeated. C again functioned on the mental scale at the superior level. Her best functioning was on Naming three objects at the 24 month level, and Naming the watch at the fourth picture, also at the 24 month level. She was able to place six blocks in the Blue Form Board, at the 22 month level, and could name three pictures at the 22 month level. Motor functioning was also above chronological age level. She was walking up stairs with help, standing up from a supine position, standing on each foot alone, and jumping off the floor. Both Décarie scales continued to be passed at highest criterion levels. On the objectal scale when mother changed from pleasant to unpleasant expressions, C. said "naughty", suggesting she was well on the way to internalizing and identifying with the maternal figure.

At two years, C. was somewhat coquettish in her initial reactions to the examiner, and did not speak above a whisper. However, once performance tests were given, she responded with more than a whisper, and attention and cooperation were good. The examiner felt that she was less shy and more outgoing in her responses than during previous examinations. C. achieved a mental age of 2-9 and IQ of 135 on the Stanford Binet, Form L-M Intelligence test. She achieved a basal at year II-6 and a ceiling at year IV. Her highest successes were on choosing the biggest ball at year III-6, and Picture Vocabulary and Copying a Circle at year III. She was able to string beads at III but not enough to score at that level. Picture Vocabulary level was between III and III-6, and suggested well developed verbal ability. Motor skills were at about level III. Both Décarie scales continued to score at the highest criterion levels.

Although the children had been ill with a virus, and were described as feverish, C. participated in the two and a half year old testing fully. She was not as shy as during previous testings, although her shyness might have reflected itself an unwillingness to make guesses and take risks on later tests. She attained a mental age of 4-1 and a resultant IQ of 152 on the Stanford Binet, Form L-M Intelligence test. We reminded the parents that this very gifted score might be less stable at the preschool years. Her highest scores were on Aesthetic Comparison (where she kept changing her choice), Opposite Analogies, and Pictorial Likenesses and Differences at age IV-6, the latter of which is often used as a predictor for reading readiness. She passed all the tests at the III-6 level and failed all tests at the V year level. Her areas of best functioning were on verbal and nonverbal reasoning, and vocabulary. Memory was not as well developed. C. was described at this age as a "delightful two and a half year old girl who relates well and is functioning at a very superior range of intelligence". Her drawing of a person was well integrated (head, eyes, and mouth), suggesting good integration and understanding of the human percept for her age. Motor coordination was judged to be at least at the three year level, although she showed some inexperience in holding the pencil.

C. was every eager to do the testing at age three, and she was the least restless of the triplets at this testing. She was considerably less shy. She conversed during the test period and she found it hard to wait her turn. She also seemed to know her own mind very well, and asked about toys in the box. Her attention was harder to hold on the Rorschach ink blot test, where she was unwilling to make a guess on several of the cards. This pattern was less noticeable on the Binet.

On the latter test, she obtained a mental age of 4-6 and IQ of 140, lower than the previous testing, but this was felt to be more related to the instability of preschool age scores. Her basal was at year IV, and ceiling where all tests were failed was at year VI. She remembered only two of three commissions at IV-6, the only item failed at year IV-6. Her highest success was on Pictorial Similarities and Differences at year V. These findings suggested unusually strong ability in reasoning. C. continued to show some difficulty in holding a pencil. Her human figure drawing included a head, and some parts of the body, not fully integrated.

C's reluctance to take a guess or to take risks on the Rorschach ambiguous ink blots resulted in a small number of responses. Her responses suggested that she was engaged in age appropriate tasks of self individuation and identity. There were some fears, but she was also extremely stimulated by the color of the cards. There seemed to be a growth spurt in her wish to make social emotional contact with others. There was more of an active-passive conflict, which was interpreted to be an emergence from her more previously shy and withdrawn state of a year ago. The examiner thought her last response of a frog jumping over a rainbow was extremely adorable and represented some creativity and a very happy, cheerful disposition,—"a happy outgoing child".

This child was one of a set of high birth weight triplets. She functioned above age level from the age of 3 months, with above average functioning by 9 months. By 15 months she was saying two word sentences, naming two objects and one picture, and pointing to the parts of a doll (19.1 month level). She was saying 22 words at that time. By age two and a half she was functioning in the gifted range of verbal intelligence. Motor functioning was above average.

Her object constancy and objectal scores correlated highly with this verbal spurt. At the age of 3 months, she attained 3 month level on the objectal scale, and no score on the object constancy scale. At 6 months this reversed itself, and she attained 9 month level on the object constancy scale and 5 month level on the objectal scale. At 9 months she attained the 11-12 month criterion level on the object constancy scale and 9 month level on the objectal scale. She reached highest criterion levels on both scales by 12 months of age (18-20 months on object constancy and 15-17 months on the objectal scale). There seemed to be a birth weight effect asserting itself in the development of this child.

Boy, A. A. was described as a sturdy, well developed infant two days short of his three month birthday. On the mental scale, his highest pass was at 3.8 months for carrying the ring to his mouth. He also fingered hands in play, followed a ball visually across a table, reached for the dangling ring, and engaged in simple play with a rattle. On the motor scale, he could balance his head, and sit with support. He also turned from his side to his back and was able to elevate himself by his arms. Motor functioning was average for this term baby. Object constancy had not yet developed, but on the objectal scale he was functioning at three months. He responded to the feeding situation, and reacted to both mother and examiner with smiling and cooing, indiscriminately. He could be comforted when crying by the seeing and talking mother, but not by the unseen mother.

A. at six months was a large, extremely vigorous six month infant, who was the most easily frustrated of the triplets, and least able to go from one test item to the other. Mental functioning was advanced and increased over the three month testing. He passed all tests through the 6.2 month level (playful response to mirror), and passed vocalizing four syllables, pulling string adaptively to secure the ring, cooperating in games, ringing bell purposively, and saying dada, all at the seven month level. The passing items were all social, language, and imitative skills. Motor development was normative, although not advanced. The items added since the three month testing related to greater prehensive ability, ability to turn over, and beginning ability to maintain a seated position. There were no observed specific difficulties with motor functions. Object constancy was developed to the six to nine month level. A. was able to search for a ball in a new place, and he could reconstruct an invisible whole from a visible fraction. He responded at the nine month level on the objectal scale. He did not discriminate mother and stranger in a social situation. However, he did cease crying with the voice of mother, and he reacted pleasurably to play of the mother, and negatively to an interruption and negatively to the loss of a toy.

A. is again described as a vigorous baby at nine months, who was easily frustrated. He interacted engagingly with his mother, and was most interested in the test material. He performed again well above his chronological age level on the mental scale. His highest successes were on jabbering expressively at the 12.0 month level, and uncovering a Blue Box, at the 12.0 month level. His earliest failure was uncovering a toy at 8.1 months and fingering holes in a peg board at 8.9 months.

A. functioned at Criterion 4 on the Décarie objectal scale. He reacted positively to mother's play and negatively to the loss of a toy. This item is at the nine month level. On the object constancy scale, he found the object under one screen, but not under two. His failure to uncover the toy on the Bayley suggested this ability was emerging. However, on the Décarie scale he scored at the eight to ten month level.

At 12 months, A. continued to be a very vigorous baby, who was easily frustrated. He was teething during this testing, and most materials were put to his mouth first, making numerous items difficult to administer. It was felt that the test score at this time was an underestimate, since he mouthed items rather than using them adaptively. There was a drop in mental index of 14 points from the previous testing. His highest successes were on using gestures to make wants known at the 14.6 month level, and saying two words at the 14.2 level. At that time, he was saying, baba, mama, dada, and bye bye. His lowest failure was on holding the crayon adaptively, as he put it in his mouth.

The motor index was also reduced about 16 points. He was the only one of the triplets who was walking but could not be interested in using the pull toy or walking sideways or backwards. His highest successes were standing up from a supine position, and throwing a ball. He had midline skill, and did seem to be in a gross motor spurt.

He succeeded at the 18-20 month level on the object constancy scale, finding the hidden object under three screens. This suggested again that the mental scores were an underestimate. He reached Criterion 6 on the objectal scale at the 15-17 month level. He responded to both a request and a prohibition. It was noted at this time that he would need help in developing more delay as he grew older, as "he may be a very active and highly forceful infant".

A. received a new examiner at 15 months. He was described as "a very outgoing child, approaching new tasks with a high level of activity and often with delight and enthusiasm". However, he is also described as willful and showing negativistic or oppositional behavior in refusing particular tasks, sometimes throwing them violently on the floor. He worked diligently and persistently with a high level of concentration for a short while. However, if he did not succeed within a fairly short time, he quickly lost interest in the task and the examiner found it generally impossible to reinterest him. He was described as social and with little wariness of strangers, so that the examiner did not attribute his behavior to the change of examiners. He was excited by the new materials, and he often leaned over and attempted to secure various toys from the examiner's table. However, "while he is delightful and appealing, he is also stubborn and can protest vigorously when his wishes are not gratified".

Mental development improved since the last testing by about 10 points. He was most advanced in his ability to discriminate forms and to place them in appropriate openings, at the 21.2 month level. His earliest failure was at the 12.4 month level, dangling a ring by a string, because of refusal. He was able to use words and gestures to make wants known, but did not name objects or discriminate them by pointing. He was saying the following words: bye bye, dada, mama, hi, boo, all gone, birdie, up, down, neigh, moo, no, cook cook, and car. Some of his earliest failures that may have been refusals were building a tower with cubes or putting cubes in a cup (at 13.8 and 14.3 months). His first failure that did not seem to be a result of refusal was placing pegs in a pegboard at 16.4 months.

Motor development was average. A. was able to walk in all directions and to stand on one foot with help. He did not walk up and down stairs with help. Objectally, he responded differentially to a threatening vs. surprised maternal expression, but did not imitate hand clapping. He passed the object constancy scale at the highest criterion, 18-20 month level, finding the object under three screens. The examiner commented on his use of "no" as a normative stage of development, which "can best be dealt with by consistent and firm limits, along with encouragement of independent efforts".

A.'s behavior during the 18 month examination was described as improved. He was somewhat shy and hesitant at first, different from his enthusiasm of the previous testing, and he consistently refused items having to do with blocks. He warmed up and worked persistently and well, but frequent interventions were needed to sustain his attention. He was distractible and interrupted testing to talk to mother. He spoke in two word sentences, for example saying "man working" about a man viewed outside the window who was working. The examiner reported a stronger frustration tolerance and better impulse control. He did become irritable after forty five minutes but calmed down when juice was given. He also became upset at one point when mother left the room.

On the Bayley scales, he achieved a superior score on the mental and motor scales, mental being higher. He was most advanced in his ability to name and point to objects and pictures, at the 25.2 month level. His earliest failure was at the 16.7 month level, because of refusal to build a tower with three cubes. He also failed such timed tasks as the peg board. He imitated a vertical and horizontal stroke at 24 months, but did not find the hidden object (19.7 months) or discriminate between three objects (23.4 months). Motor development was also above developmental expectations. He was able to stand alone on each foot, jump off the floor, and jump from the bottom step (24.8 months). Object relations was at the highest criterion: he had already passed the response to request and prohibition at 15-17 months, and at this time added the differential response to maternal expression and the imitation of hand clapping. He was noted to pat himself on the back when he coughed, also an imitation of maternal caring, suggesting good internalization of the maternal object. Object constancy continued to be passed at the highest criterion, 18-20 months, finding the object under three screens. The examiner said at this time: "Much of the oppositionality and negativism which characterized D. at 15 months is no longer evident at 18 months. A. is becoming more able to delay gratification and shows signs of internalizing parental caregiving. He continues to be an active, vigorous child who easily displays his emotions."

At age two, A. was described as entering an oppostional phase, that the examiner explained in terms of his age. Testing was somewhat hampered by this, as he was quite active and tended to become stubborn and to refuse tasks. He was demanding, exploring new toys often to the neglect of tasks presented to him. This occurred most often when he was frustrated with a task. When he was interested in a task, however, he responded readily with little hesitation. He was also responsive to encouragement and praise. His attention span was short at times, but again not felt to be inappropriate for a two year old. He was eager to end the session and was allowed to complete the tests while standing.

He obtained a mental age of 2-9 and IQ of 135 on the Stanford Binet, Form L-M Intelligence test. Basal was at II and ceiling at IV. The oppositionality did not substantially interfere with his performance. He failed items gradually, but with failures, he refused tasks frequently. The earliest failure occurred in block building and in obeying simple commands. It was felt that these were refusals. Language development was particularly advanced. He had some three word sentences and the vocabulary and verbal fluency of a three year old. He also passed one comprehension item at the III-6 level. He had the most difficulty with items requiring visual motor abilities, such as stringing beads and block building, at the III year level. The objectal and object constancy tests were passed at the highest criterion level at the previous testing. At this time, the examiner felt that the oppositionality and demandingness were not unusual for a two year old, but that the lowered frustration tolerance was "somewhat lower than expected". The examiner recommended consistent limits along with warmth and empathy.

The two and a half year old testing of A. occurred under difficult circumstances. A. had a fever of 103 degrees, and he was quite difficult to test. His attention span was adequate for the first ten minutes, and he persisted on difficult tasks with encouragement. After this, his attention span was quite short, he refused many items, and did not persevere in the face of even slight difficulty. Otherwise, he was outgoing and confident socially, when he was not required to perform tasks. He offered the examiner crackers, smiled, spoke her name, and was charming and engaging. Problem solving was often ineffective, however. He reacted strongly to failure by withdrawing and increasing his activity, refusing tasks, and giving up easily. He required constant limit setting, but did not respond well to those given by either examiner or mother.

Stanford Binet, Form L-M functioning was below the level of the previous testing. He obtained a mental age of 2-6 and IQ of 126. His basal was at II-6 and a ceiling was estimated at year VI (because of increased activity and refusals). He failed the visual motor items presented at III and continued to fail all items requiring visual motor integration. Fine motor coordination was notably poor. On the other hand, general comprehension and reasoning items requiring verbal abilities were passed through the V year level. It should be noted that the perceptual motor abilities were poor only relative to his advanced verbal abilities, but not below age level. Short attention span was noted particularly on tasks requiring that he remember a hidden object for 10 seconds. The examiner felt that the illness contributed to D.'s difficulties during this testing, but that the test patterning suggested a needed follow up with further testing to determine whether there was a relative perceptual motor problem.

A. was initially cheerful and smiling, but slightly apprehensive about the three year testing. He was tested this time without mother present, although she was available in the next room. He refused the first task of drawing a person, saying he couldn't do it, but with encouragement he scribbled what he said were an ear, a mouth, etc. He enjoyed the encouragement and praise, but his pattern of refusal of tasks continued, and hesitancy was replaced with oppositionality. He particularly did not like the visuo motor tasks. He was active and ran out of the room to establish contact with his mother, and also called to her while being tested. He responded better to limits when given choices, than he had in the last testing session. He was social, and his language was very well developed, saying, "That's an American flag, you pledge allegiance to the flag". He was curious about the co-examiner in the next room, possibly afraid that he was missing something that he could not have. When mother joined the last part of the session, it was when the tasks were becoming more difficult. His attention span was short, he was easily distracted, and he did not persist on the more difficult tasks. He tended to give up rather than try, although he could do the tasks if he persisted. A. related well to the adult examiner, but was not confident of his abilities. He needed much reassurance and distrusted his abilities. He was emotionally dependent and did not persist in problem solving. He showed a low frustration tolerance, withdrawal, oppositionality, and a high activity level.

On the Stanford Binet, Form L-M Intelligence test, he obtained a mental age of 4-1 and IQ of 128 at age three. His basal level was at III, and the ceiling was at V. His first failure was in distinguishing relative sizes of circles, a visual motor test at III-6. The IV and IV-6 year items that he failed tapped memory, concentration, and comprehension abilities. He passed all items dealing with vocabulary, verbal fluency, judgment, and reasoning to the V year level. Thus, his strongest abilities centered around verbal-conceptual development and logical reasoning. Relatively weaker were comprehension, attentional and memory abilities, and visual motor organization. His fine motor coordination on the human figure drawing was also relatively poor in light of his superior functioning in other areas. However, all abilities were at or above age level.

A.'s Rorschach yielded II responses which showed ability to integrate details into wholes and his perceptions were accurate. His responses included animals and human-like figures, indicating adequate social orientation and the beginnings of internalization of parental norms and societal values. However, he did not respond to the emotional aspects of the stimuli. The examiner suggested that he might experience feelings which were difficult for him to express or to integrate into a positive, comprehensive sense of self. He showed indications of self-doubt and some shame, and some suggestion that he questions his ability to function autonomously. Thus, "he may seek more reassurance and express more dependency than would be expected". Because of the interference with autonomous functioning, his doubts about his abilities and needs for reassurance and encouragement, it was suggested at this time that some work with parents might be helpful to facilitate the establishment of a more positive sense of self worth.

This high birth weight triplet showed average mental and motor functioning until 9 months of age, some increment then with a relative decrement at 12 months. By 15 months mental development was more stable and above average and motor development was average. The examiner was beginning to see poor frustration tolerance and a short attention span. At 18 months he was saying two word sentences and mental functioning was superior, and remained so for the remainder of this series. However, at the 24 month testing the examiner was beginning to see some fine motor coordination difficulties, continuing to be accompanied by poor frustration tolerance and impulsivity, for which he was later treated.

As with the previous infants, no object constancy score was obtained at three months, and an objectal score at three months was obtained. The object constancy and objectal scores were at the same level at six months, and by 9 months the score was higher on the objectal scale. At 12 months he had reached criterion level on both scales.

SUMMARY AND DISCUSSION

These detailed clinical vignettes were given to more clearly demonstrate the complexity and variability of functioning that might be obscured by the overall statistical results. By including low birthweight, middle birthweight, and high birthweight infants, we hoped to clarify and distinguish between birthweight effects and the other less tangible variables, such as socioeconomic status and more subtle attachment and personality factors.

We can see from low birth weight A that the superior mental functioning outcome could not have been predicted from her very low birthweight status. Low birthweight without accompanying neurological complications did not predict outcome in this sample. Also, we have seen that some of the infants of middle and high birthweight also had at least subtle neurological indicators, and/or personality functioning that suggested this (middle birth weight B and high birth weight A).

In our summary for each infant presented, we have also traced their object constancy and objectal development in the hope that this would clarify their attachment status through the developmental period presented. These sequential findings for individual infants are obscured in the correlational tables. All infants in this example began with no object constancy score at 3 months, but with an objectal score at the 3 month level. The objectal scores were advanced over object constancy scores for the low and middle birthweight children, with increases in mental scores accompanying a spurt in objectal score for those examples. When there was a décalage in the opposite direction (object constancy advanced over objectal development), as in middle birth weight B, there was also relative difficulty in the development of language skills with relatively better perceptual skills. This child had prehension and midline difficulties, which may be related to this relatively delayed language development and may represent a neurological effect (see Chapter 9 on language development).

Another interesting finding in these more detailed observations is that both high birthweight youngsters showed some fluctuation from the 3 month level, where objectal scores were higher, to the 12 month level, when they both attained highest level on both scales. In these two infants combined birthweight and socioeconomic effects seem to be important.

The overall impression is of décalage of objectal score over object constancy from early on with objectal measures being highly correlated with mental spurt at the lower birthweight levels, and both scores showing an increase prior to the mental spurt at the higher birthweight levels. If we can consider the objectal score to most represent the attachment to the mother, we may say that there was sufficient attachment for all of the infants in this example section to achieve average to superior mental status by age 3, or earlier.

REFERENCES

Korner, A. F., Brown Jr., B. W., Dimiceli, S., Forrest, T., Stevenson, D. K., Lane, N. M., Constantinou, J., & Thom, V. A. 1989. Stable Individual Differences in Developmentally Changing Preterm Infants. *Child Development*, 60 (2), 502–513.

Landry, S. H., Chapieski, L., Fletcher, J. M., & Denson, S. 1988. Three-Year Outcomes for Low Birth Weight Infants: Differential Effects of Early Medical Complications. *Journal of Pediatric Psychology*, 13 (3), 317–328.

Piper, M. C., Mazer, B., Silver, K. M., & Ramsay, M. 1988. Resolution of Neurological Symptoms in High-risk Infants during the first two years of life. *Developmental Medicine and Child Neurology*, 30 (1), 26–36.

CHAPTER 7

How Mother and Baby Love Influenced Development

One of the unique characteristics of the multiple birth event is that the infant and child will necessarily be cared for by multiple caregivers, particularly in the early months of life. A complexity in our understanding of their early development is the role that this multiple caretaking plays in influencing the early (and later) development of these children. We asked ourselves the question of whether the multiple care taking situation required by the mutliple birth resulted in special interferences early in the social experience of these infants, particularly in the attachment to the mother. Such interference would have implications for the sufficient development of a mother infant bond and the resultant effects on object constancy, and object relations (also referred to as attachment) beyond the effects attributed to low birth weight and prematurity.

The object concept relates to the regular development of the concept of "object" when things are "conceived as permanent, substantial, external to the self, and firm in existence even though they do not directly affect perception" (Décarie, 1965:29). We are using the term object relations after Décarie, who defines its general meaning as "the affective tie which a subject establishes with an object" (Décarie, 1965). The concept of attachment has been developed by Bowlby (1969) in its more ethological sense that the infant has a bias toward attaching himself especially to one figure, usually the mother.

Bowlby (1969) differs from Freud's concept of the mother infant relationship as based on the child's physiological need for food and warmth, which Bowlby calls the secondary drive hypothesis. His theory "postulates that the child's tie to his mother is a product of the activity of a number of behavioural systems that have proximity to mother as a predictable outcome" (1969, p.179). He states that the function of these behavioral systems is for protection against predators, and calls this tie to the mother "attachment".

Ainsworth (1982) describes four behavioral systems that interact to form the baby's attachment behavior: attachment, wariness/fear, affiliation or sociability, and exploration. She believes that it is the pattern of these behavioral systems rather than any specific behaviors that determine the baby's attachment behavior. Because the baby's attachment to the mother is most threatened when separated from the mother, she developed a method of studying the baby's attachment to the mother through the "strange situation". This involves seven episodes of separation from the mother and introduction of a strange person. She has been able to identify three patterns of attachment to the mother: securely attached, anxiously-avoidant, and anxiously-ambivalent. She notes that a child's attachment to his mother undergoes developmental changes, and may also be subject to environmental or life stresses.

Ainsworth (1982) also discusses the concept of an hierarchy of attachment figures. She quotes Bowlby (1969) as saying that a child is likely to be especially attached to one principal figure and called the other persons to whom he might be attached subsidiary or secondary attachment figurtes, and that the child when distressed or ill is more likely to go to that principal figure, the mother. There have been few research reports on attachment to figures other than the mother. Ainsworth (1982) reports that studies of the father-child attachment using the strange situation method have shown that a child securely attached to the mother was equally likely to be securely or anxiously attached to the father. There remains the question of other figures, the nature of a baby's attachment to them, whether other attachments can substitute for the attachment to the mother, and whether these attachments are equal to each other or stand in some hierarchical arrangement of greater or lesser capacity to substitute for the mother.

Décarie (1965) found a very close relationship between object relations and object constancy, and a high correlation of both to mental development, as measured by the Griffith scales. We were interested in whether these findings would be differentially influenced by the mutliple birth situation and the multiple caretaking environment of multiple birth infants. A positive décalage (Bell, 1970), that is, object relations advanced over object constancy, might indicate greater attachment to the mother, and to predict greater stranger anxiety (Brossard, 1974). A negative décalage (object constancy advanced over object relations) might indicate some delay and/or interference with the mother-infant bond. With the presence of many nonspecific attachments, it could be hypothesized that object relations (that is, specific attachment to the mother) would be delayed relative to object constancy in the multiple birth infant.

Although there is little direct research on this issue concerning multiple birth infants, there is some discussion in the attachment literature concerning when specific attachment to the mother occurs, and whether multiple caretaking affects this specific attachment (Ainsworth, 1963; Schaffer, 1963). Schaffer posits that there is a period of indiscriminate relatedness before there is specific attachment to the mother. Ainsworth states that the attachment is always to the mother first. Our infants are more like Ainsworth's Ganda infants where there were often multiple caretakers. She found that the multiple caretaking situation did not interfere with the specific attachment to the mother. Schaffer's argument is that it does not matter what parenting figures are available in the early months of the infant's life providing there is early social stimulation. Following this, the infant seeks out the specific attachment to the mother, and there are often other figures to whom they also make a specific attachment. Following Ainsworth, we should expect that our multiply cared for babies would have as strong a specific attachment to the mother as singleton children who have been cared for mainly by mother. Schaffer's hypothesis would, however, also lead us to look for specific attachments to others, as well.

Day care and kibbutz studies may have some illuminating findings with regard to these considerations. Caldwell (1970) concluded that full-time day care did not prevent children from developing attachments of normal strength to their mothers. Her infants sometimes were placed as early as six months, but more often at one year. However, Blehar (1974) found that the younger children in her group (26 months of age) were more detached following separations, while the older children (35 months of age) were anxious and ambivalent after separation. She suggests that there is a qualitative disturbance in attachment relationships, obscured in the Caldwell study because they focussed on attachment rather than on separation, and did not differentiate age levels. She emphasized the importance of the quality of mother-child relationships prior to day care, and the quality of day care itself. More recent day care literature suggests that full-time day care need not prevent children from developing attachments of normal strength to their mothers (Roopnarine & Lamb, 1978; Doyle

& Somers, 1978; Ragozin, 1980; Moskowitz, Schwarz, & Corsini, 1977; Cornelius & Denney, 1975; and Rubenstein, Pederson, & Yarrow, 1977).

An earlier preliminary report by Caldwell (1962) reported that infants from monomatric families (families in which maternal care is provided almost exclusively by mother) were rated as more affiliative and dependent and manifested more affect in interaction with their mothers than infants from polymatric families (families in which a substantial amount of maternal care is provided by one or more persons in addition to the mother).

Studies of kibbutz children reared apart from their parents in a collective setting, with varied contacts with parental figures from kibbutz and over the age range studied by us, reveal that kibbutz children obtained developmental scores that are superior to Israeli private home infants (Kohen-Raz, 1968). There was no relation between developmental quotient and frequence of caretaker change. The percentage of mothering stimulation was lower for kibbutz infants except in the first six months (Landau, 1976). However, Maccoby and Feldman (1972) found attachment patterns of kibbutz and U. S. children to be highly similar. They raise the possibility that there is a critical period before six months, during which time the mother does spend more time with her kibbutz infant. Provence and Lipton (1962) also emphasize the importance of the first year. A second possibility that Maccoby and Feldman cite is that there has to be a minimally adequate amount of contact between child and mothering object and this is an amount which both environments provide. They raise the question as to what is a "minimally adequate environment", and the possibility that it is not the quantity of mothering which is concerned but the quality of mothering. It may well be this quality of interaction between mother and child, not the sheer availability.

This hypothesis is supported by Anderson et al. (1981), who found high interactive day care centers to have children behaving more like securely attached children in the strange situation. Fox (1977) found kibbutz children to react similarly with metapelet and mother at separation, but differentially and with more upset with reunion to the metapelet. They concluded that they were more attached to mother than to the metapelet.

It is interesting at this time to refer to the 1982 followup of kibbutz children grown up (Rabin and Beit-Hallahmi, 1982). The findings showed that at the infancy stage, the kibbutz youngster showed less positive development than those in the control group, but that at the

Table 7.1. Correlations of objectal relations scores with birth weight

Age in months	3	6	9	12	15
N	16	16	15	19	19
Correlations	.55	.60	.72	.44	.49
Mean Scores	2.31	4.25	5.40	8.79	12.53
Standard Deviations	.48	1.73	2.97	3.39	3.63
p: Level of Significance	.05	.01	.01	.05	.05

ten-year level, intellectual, ego strength, adjustment and emotional maturity tended to favor the kibbutz. The same trend was noted in adolescent findings. There were no significant differences found in adjustment levels between the two groups.

We might hypothesize that the capacity for object relations and/or mother infant attachment would be expected to precede object constancy, or at least not lag behind, in multiple birth infants, should Ainsworth be correct. However, if Caldwell's preliminary findings with regard to polymatric families is correct, then there might be an attachment lag, that is a negative décalage.

The additional effect of their status as premature infants may be compensated by the tendency of mothers of prematures to be more highly interactive with their infants (Minde, Perrotta, & Hellmann, 1988). Easterbrook (1989) has found that preterm infants do form secure attachments to their mothers.

The results to be presented in this chapter will examine the scores from the objectal and object constancy scales and their relationship to birthweight (and the related factor of prematurity) on mental and motor development. At a later time we may also want to return to these early infancy findings to consider whether there has been more long term effects of prematurity and the multiple birth situation on later emotional and personality functioning.

RESULTS

Objectal scores were higher than object constancy scores at 3 and 6 months. (See Tables 7.1 and 7.2). This discrepancy (décalage) in favor of object relations scores lasted longer for the low birth weight children, and those who reached the highest criterion on the object constancy scale earlier were of higher birth weight. Note that the correlations of birth weight with the objectal relations scores are significant between 3 and 15 months (p .05, .01, .01, .05, .05). The

Table 7.2. Correlations of object constancy scores with birth weight

Age in months	6	9	12	15	18
N	16	15	19	19	17
Correlation	.68	.76	.75	.67	.63
Mean Scores	2.25	5.53	9.74	12.63	15.29
Standard Deviations	2.57	3.74	3.65	3.64	3.92
p: Level of Significance	.01	.01	.01	.01	.01

correlations between birth weight and object constancy scores are significant between 6 and 18 months (p .01 for all ages). It is also interesting to note that once there was a shift in décalage at 9 months, the increase in score for object constancy measures continued until the criterion was reached by all subjects, by 24 months.

Objectal scores were correlated with MDI (mental development) smoothed adjusted scores at 6, 9, and 15 months (p .05, .01, .01); and object constancy with MDI smoothed adjusted scores at 9, 15, and 18 months (p .01, .05, .01). (See Tables 7.3 and 7.4). Objectal scores were correlated with PDI (motor development) smoothed adjusted scores at 3, 9, and 15 months (p .05, .01, and .05); and object constancy with PDI smoothed adjusted scores at 9, and 18 months (p .01). Again there is a trend for the objectal scores to be correlated at the earlier ages, and the object constancy scale to be correlated at the later ages. (See Tables 7.5 and 7.6). Object constancy and objectal scores correlated with each other between 6 months and 15 months (p .05, .01, .01, .05). (See Table 7.7.)

Table 7.3. Correlations of objectal scores with smoothed adjusted mental scale scores

Age in months	3	6	9	12	15
N	16	16	12	19	19
Correlations	.42	.55	.76	.15	.61
Means of Mental Score	115	115	98	100	106
Standard Deviations	16.06	17.56	18.87	18.30	22.99
Mean Objectal Scores	2.31	4.25	5.75	8.79	12.53
Standard Deviations	.48	1.73	3.17	3.39	3.63
p: Level of Significance	NS	.05	.01	NS	.01

Table 7.4. Correlation of object constancy scores with smoothed adjusted mental scale scores

Age in months	9	12	15	18
N	12	19	19	17
Correlations	.85	.39	.49	.72
Means of Mental Scores	98	100	106	106
Standard Deviations	18.87	18.30	22.99	21.74
Mean Object Constancy Scores	5.00	10.26	12.95	15.53
Standard Deviations	3.84	3.49	3.27	3.48
p: Level of Significance	.01	NS	.05	.01

Table 7.5. Correlation of objectal scores with smoothed adjusted motor scale scores

Age in months	3	6	9	12	15
N	16	16	12	19	19
Correlations	−.53	.12	.86	.20	.51
Means of Motor Scores	129	111	97	98	96
Standard Deviations	20.03	21.77	18.95	20.20	13.50
Mean Objectal Scores	2.31	4.25	5.75	8.79	12.53
Standard Deviations	.48	1.73	3.17	3.39	3.63
p: Level of Significance	.05	NS	.01	NS	.05

Table 7.6. Correlation of object constancy scores with smoothed adjusted motor scale scores

Age in Months	6	9	12	15	18
N	16	12	19	19	19
Correlations	−.38	.79	.16	.37	.59
Means of Motor Scores	111	97	98	96	99
Standard Deviations	21.77	18.95	20.20	13.50	15.71
Means of Object Constancy Scores	2.25	5.00	10.26	12.95	15.53
Standard Deviations	2.57	3.84	3.49	3.27	3.48
p: Level of Significance	NS	.01	NS	NS	.01

Table 7.7. Correlation of objectal and object constancy scales

Age in months	6	9	12	15
N	16	15	19	19
Correlations	.49	.62	.70	.47
p: Level of Significance	.05	.01	.01	.05

DISCUSSION

Although objectal development was delayed as compared to babies of normal weight and gestation, it preceded the development of object constancy in the earliest months of life. If one considers that the object relations measure is related to the development of person permanence (Bell, 1970), it suggests that for our infants in a multiple caretaking situation, the specific attachment to the mothering figure was not impaired. Ainsworth (1963) reports that her detailed findings suggest that "a child cared for by several caretakers can, and frequently does, form as secure an attachment to one figure, his mother, as a child who has a more exclusive relationship with one figure . . . given an opportunity to do so, an infant will seek an attachment with one figure, the person primarily responsible for his care, even though there are several persons available as caretakers". Lamb (1978) has explored the relationship of the infant with father as well as mother, and has indicated that the infant can form a differential relationship with either, depending on which relationship is most precedent in time and the nature of the relationship. Marvin (1978) found that contact and physical interaction are more important in the formation of a specific attachment than feeding, among the Hausa infants of Nigeria.

Given the hypothesis that it is not the extent or amount of specific relationship with the mother, and the quality of that relationship rather than the general availability of the mother, one might posit that there was an adequate amount of mothering available to these infants. They did seek out a specific relationship to the mother. However, it is possible that rather than heightened objectal relationships, it means lowered object constancy in those first few months. This would mean that there was an intellectual delay consequent to the low birth weight and prematurity of the infants, and that it takes some time for intellectual skills and object constancy to catch up to the relatedness measures. However, in both our study and in that of Caldwell (1970) on day care infants, the better developed infants tended also to be more strongly attached to their mothers, i.e. to have higher object relations measures.

There seems to be a close correspondence between intellectual development and the object relations scale measures (at 6, 9, and 15 months) and between object constancy measures and mental development (at 9, 15, and 18 months). Object constancy and objectal relations scores are significantly correlated with each other at 6, 9, 12, and 15 months. There is a suggestion that at the early ages objectal development is more related to intellectual development, while later there is a closer correspondence with object constancy as a forerunner of cognitive capacities.

Nelson (1979) also found a relationship between object constancy and Bayley scores; low scores on the Bayley were related to delays in achievement of "object permanence" for low SES subjects. These observations suggest that when object relations achieve some more mature level, both object constancy measures and intellectual development increase, and other factors such as the social environment, SES, and possibly the stimulation of other siblings may more clearly influence intellectual development beyond birth weight and other maturational effects. Sigman and Parmalee (1979) found that inclusion of home observation measures improved prediction of high risk status in infants and concluded that the interaction of the caregiver and infant was highly important for outcome.

REFERENCES

Ainsworth, M. D. 1963. The development of mother-infant interaction among the Ganda. In B. Foss (Ed.) *Determinants of Infant behavior*. II. London: Methuen.

Ainsworth, M. D. 1969. Object relations, dependency and attachment: a theoretical review of the infant-mother relationship. *Child Development*. 40: 969–1025.

Ainsworth, M. D. 1982. Attachment, Retrospect and Prospect. In C. M. Parks & J. Stevenson-Hinde (Eds.) *The Place of Attachment in Human Behavior*. New York: Basic Books, Inc., Publishers.

Anderson, W. A., Nagle, R. J., Roberts, W. A. and Smith, J. W. 1981. Attachment to substitute caregivers as a function of center quality and caregiver involvement. *Child Development*. 52: 53–61.

Bell, S. M. 1970. The development of the concept of object as related to infant-mother attachment. *Child Development*. 41: 291–311.

Blehar, M. D. 1974. Anxious attachment and defensive reactions associated with day care. *Child Development*. 45: 683–692.

Bowlby, J. 1969. Attachment And Loss. Volume 1. *Attachment*. New York: Basic Books, Inc., Publishers.

Brossard, M. D. 1974. II. The infant's conception of object permanence and his reactions to strangers. In T. G. Décarie (Ed.) *The infant's reactions to strangers*. New York: International Universities Press, Inc.

Caldwell, B., Hersher, L., Lipton, E., Richmond, J. B., Stern, G., Eddy, E. J., and Drachman, R. 1962. Mother-infant interaction in monomatric and polymatric families. *American Journal of Orthopsychiatry*. 32: 340–341.

Caldwell, B., Wright, C. M., Honig, A. S., and Tannenbaum, J. 1970. Infant day care and attachment. *American Journal of Orthopsychiatry*. 40: 397–412.

Cornelius, S. W., and Denny, N. W. 1975. Dependency in day-care and home-care children. *Developmental Psychology*. II:575–582.

Décarie, T. G. 1965. *Intelligence and affectivity in early childhood*. New York: International Universities Press, Inc.

Doyle, A. B., and Somers, K. 1978. The effects of group and family day care on infant attachment behaviours. *Canadian Journal of Behavioral Science*. 10, 1: 38–45.

Easterbrook, M. A. 1989. Quality of attachment to mother and to father: Effects of Perinatal Risk Status. *Child Development*, 60 (4), 825–830.

Fox, N. 1977. Attachment of kibbutz infants to mother and metapelet. *Child Development*. 48: 1228–1239.

Kohen-Raz, R. 1968. Mental and motor development of kibbutz, institutionalized and home-reared infants in Israel. *Child Development*. 39: 489–514.

Lamb, M. E. 1978. Qualitative aspects of mother- and father-infant attachments. *Infant Behavior and Development*. 1: 265–275.

Landau, H. 1976. Extent that the mother represents the social stimulation to which the infant is exposed: findings from a cross-cultural study. *Developmental Psychology*. 12: 399–405.

Maccoby, E. E., and Feldman, S. S. 1972. Mother-attachment and stranger-reactions in the third year of life. *Monographs of the Society for Research in Child Development*. 37:1.

Marvin, R. S., Van Devender, T., Iwanaga, M. I., LeVine, S., and LeVine, R. A. 1978. Infant-caregiver attachment among the Hausa of Nigeria. In H. McGurk (Ed.) *Ecological factors in human development*. Amsterdam: North-Holland Publishing Co.

Minde, K., Perrotta, M., & Hellmann, J. 1988. Impact of delayed development in premature infants on mother-infant interaction: A prospective investigation. *Journal of Pediatrics*, 112, 136–142.

Moskowitz, D. D., Schwarz, J. C., and Corsini, D. A. 1977. Initiating day care at three years of age: Effects on attachment. *Child Development*. 48: 1271–1276.

Nelson, M. N. 1979. Bayley developmental assessments of low birthweight infants. In T. M. Field (Ed.) *Infants born at risk*. New York: SP Medical and Scientific Books.

Provence, S., and Lipton, R. C. 1962. *Infants in institutions*. New York: International Universities Press, Inc.

Rabin, A. I., and Beit-Hallahmi. 1982. *Twenty years later. Kibbutz children grown up*. New York: Springer.

Ragozin, A. S. 1980. Attachment behavior of day-care children: Naturalistic and laboratory observations. *Child Development*. 51: 409–415.

Roopnarine, J. L., and Lamb, M. E. 1978. The effects of day care on attachment and exploratory behavior in a strange situation. *Merrill-Palmer Quarterly*. 24: 85–95.

Rubenstein, J. L., Pedersen, F. A., and Yarrow, L. J. 1977. What happens when mother is away: A comparison of mothers and substitute caregivers. *Developmental Psychology*. 13: 529–530.

Schaffer, H. R. 1963. Some issues for research in the study of attachment behavior. In B. Foss (Ed.) *Determinants of Infant Behavior. II*. London: Methuen.

Schaffer, H. R., and Emerson, P. E. 1964. The development of social attachments in infancy. *Monographs of the Society for Research in Child Development*. 29:3.

Sigman, M., and Parmalee, A. H. 1979. Longitudinal evaluation of the pre-term infant. In T. M. Field. (Ed.) *Infants born at risk*. New York: SP Medical and Scientific Books.

CHAPTER 8

Parenting and Interventions

Two characteristics of this sample provided some interesting concerns regarding the parenting of the cohorts. The first, the multiple birth status and inevitable multiple parenting that would result was addressed more globally in the previous chapter. The other issue which cross cut this one is that of the prematurity and low birth weight itself that existed in three of the cohorts, thus affecting thirteen of the nineteen children in the core sample.

In four of the families, hospital discharge was delayed, the least amount of time in hospital being from 5–10 days for these cohorts. The literature has questioned whether there is a critical period for bonding, with recommendations that there be early opportunities for contact in hospital. Goldberg's review (1983) suggests that the present studies are inconclusive, and she advises caution in assuming that if there is a delay in contact, necessarily deleterious effects will occur.

Probably more emphasis might be placed upon the nature of the interactions once the infants are joined with parental figures. Reviews of the literature on the mother-infant dyads in preterm infants and high risk infants suggest that the early care of these infants is problematic. The infants are characterized by delays in milestones, and less active in response to the parents or caregiver; and the parents tend either to be less physically available to them, or less sensitive to them or less synchronous in their response to them. Field (1979) adds that the infants are less responsive to the parents because of the overstimulation that the parent presents to them in an attempt to activate them. Stern and Karraker (1988) report on tendencies for mothers to stereotype prematures and to respond to them as delayed.

It is important to note that most recent literature suggests, however, that after a while (8–10 months), the early disparities in infant-parent reactions reported apparently disappear. Whether these disappear because of fading away, or improvement in dyad relationships, or failure in the measurements used, Holmes et al. (1984) do not know.

In our parents, we noted a slump or depressive reaction across all families at the nine month point, and counselling needed to occur at that time to relieve what we called "battle fatigue." This seems to coincide with the time reported here that the differences between full term and preterm infants diminished or were not measurable. It suggests that our parents were in an intense struggle until this time to cope with both the developmental delays of their infants, where present; and with the multiple children. As reported in an earlier chapter, our families uniformly reported the first year to be one of stress for them, emotionally and physically (and sometimes economically, adding further stress). Trause and Kramer (1984) report on a middle income sample of parents of low risk youngsters that parents were extremely distressed following a premature birth. However, they also report that the premature baby's mothers were less distressed by the time the babies returned home, than the full term mothers, having had interventions and care through hospital interventions, and seven months later there were no differences between mothers of preterm and full term infants. They attribute these findings to the large amount of contact between parents and infants; the economic and social stability of the families; and the relatively good health of the infants. This sample seems very similar to that of ours following discharge.

Feinstein (1984) reports that in recent times the birth of multiples has more positive implications and parents do not see their parenting tasks as particularly different from singleton births. As we have noted, our parents sought these births knowing in advance that the chances were the births would be multiple since they were conceived on the basis of fertility drugs; quoting from Feinstein: "Early diagnosis, high quality prenatal care, and techniques that avoid premature birth through the use of labor prevention medications has resulted in higher birth weight multiples." However, he does report the problems noted above, the economic and physical exhaustion stress.

In our sample, the interventions of counselling at the point of exhaustion and stress, and the ongoing contact with the investigators aided in the reduction of stress with constant feedback on the ongoing development of the infants and children. Our reference to the social support system in an earlier chapter is of importance here. All parents reported that they would have liked more time alone; and all reported that their spouses were of considerable help to them.

Investigators have demonstrated the importance of father relationships (Lamb, 1978; Levy-Shiff, Sharir, & Mogilner, 1989), and indicate that the nature of the interaction between infants and caretaker will determine the quality of that relationship for fathers as well as mothers. It was our impression that the nature of the multiple birth situation was such that it pulled for considerable father involvement in the caretaking of our children. All parents reported this factor in their being able to survive that first year. Also, throughout the study, the fathers have been very active in contributing to the study. Crnic et al. (1983) have recently studied the issue of social supports and its effects on parenting attitudes, mother-infant interaction, and infant development, with positive results for premature infants in particular.

In addition to spouses and the extended families in our cohorts, the support system always included the examiners who visited the homes in the first year every three months, and after that every six months and then yearly. Our sessions always included an informal feedback session; and a psychological and psycho-social test report. Whenever there was an emotional or social crisis, the parents called us for assistance. At times, additional testing was done to aid in school reported difficulties.

An additional influence in these families is that of the sibling status in the multiple birth situation. Our parents early reported a sibling effect in the developmental progression of their children. One child tended to lead in developmental milestones, and the others followed. The nature of twinning and its psychoanalytic meaning for ego development was also commented upon by Feinstein. Certainly having another female or male counterpart of an exact age must have far reaching effects on personality development and as an emotional and social support. We will have more to say about these effects in our later chapter on personality development.

REFERENCES

Crnic, K. A., Greenberg, M. T., Ragozin, A. S., Robinson, N. M., & Basham, R. B. 1983. Effects of stress and social support on mothers and premature and full-term infants. *Child Development*, 54: 209–217.

Feinstein, S. 1985. Multiple births and Twins. In H. I. Kaplan & B. Sadock (Eds.) *Comprehensive Textbook of Psychiatry*. Baltimore, Maryland: Williams & Wilkins.

Field, T. M. Interaction patterns of preterm and term infants. 1979. In T. M. Field, A. M. Sosek, and H. H. Shuman (Eds.) *Infants born at risk: Behavior and development*. New York: SP Medical and Scientific and Medical Books.

Goldberg, S. 1983. Parent-infant bonding: Another look. *Child Development*. 54: 1355–1382.

Holmes, D. L., Reisch, J. N., and Pasternak, J. F. 1984. Chapter 6. The high risk infant: Beyond the neonatal period. In Holmes, Reich, and Pasternak (Eds.) *The Development of infants born at risk*. Hillsdale, New Jersey: Lawrence Erlbaum Associates, Publishers.

Lamb, M. E. 1978. Qualitative aspects of mother- and father-infant attachments. *Infant Behavior and Development*. 1: 265–275.

Levy-Shiff, R., Sharir, H., and Mogilner, M. B. 1989. Mother- and Father-Preterm Infant Relationship in the Hospital Preterm Nursery. *Child Development*, 60: 93–102.

Stern, M., and Karraker, K. H. 1988. Prematurity Stereotyping by Mothers of Premature Infants. *Journal of Pediatric Psychology*. 13: 255–264.

Trause, M. A. and Kramer, L. I. 1983. The effects of premature birth on parents and their relationships. *Developmental Medicine and Child Neurology*. 25: 459–465.

CHAPTER 9

The Path to Speech and Ability

There has been considerable interest and debate over the past few decades, beginning with Wellman's famous controversey over the floating IQ, concerning the predictability of intelligence, the etiology whether nature or nature, and the earliest one can predict intellectual outcome, particularly for high risk infants.

Restructuring of the questions concerning the continuity of early behaviors of infancy with later development has led to some recent research in this area of study. Earlier research on infant measures focussed on the relationship of total developmental scores with later developmental scores. The more recent research has studied the relationship of developing specific abilities to later measures. The results of these studies have provided an interesting confirmation for the concept that there is a continuity in the development of both intellectual and language functions which can be measured early and which is predictive of later outcome (Siegel, 1979; Siegel, 1981).

Of considerable concern has been the possibility of intellectual and language delay in high risk youngsters, and not only what factors will detect those with less hopeful outcomes; but early prediction so that intervention measures can be introduced early. We have reported in an earlier chapter on the developmental outcome of our sample of multiple birth children to three years of age. In this chapter we should like to study in more detail the relationship between earlier measures and later outcome. Since we have the capability of comparing some of the same functions reported in the researches described above, it seems that we might be able to answer some of the same questions concerning continuity of development across time; and whether our early measures predicted later outcome, when specific abilities are studied rather than global measures.

The measures that were used for this comparison are described in some detail in the chapter on procedures. The comparisons for this

Table 9.1. Language Scores at $2\frac{1}{2}$ years

Range	7–19
Mean	11.47
Standard Deviation	3.84

review were between a measure of language developed from the expressive and receptive subitems of the Stanford Binet at age $2\frac{1}{2}$ (Valett, 1965), and the subscale scores of the Bayley developed by Kohen-Raz (1967). We also studied the relationship of these measures and total mental and motor scale developmental scores to Binet mental age.

RESULTS

Table 9.1 gives the range, mean and standard deviation for the language scores. Table 9.2 shows the correlations of the Kohen-Raz subscales of the Bayley with the language scores. The correlations were high and most were significant (range .61 to .84 for 6 months, .42 to .78 for 9 months, .36 to .78 at 12 months, .12 to .74 for 15 months, and .48 to .78 for 18 months).

There is a pattern of earlier scales having higher correlations at earlier ages, and later scales at later ages. For example, at 6 months the significant correlations are on eye-hand coordination, manipulation and object relations; at 9 months, manipulation, object rela-

Table 9.2. Correlations of Kohen-Raz subscales of the Bayley with total language scores on the Binet at $2\frac{1}{2}$ years

Kohen-Raz Subscales				
Eye–Hand	Manipulation	Object Relations	Imitation–Comprehension	Vocalization–Social
		6 months N=16		
.84***	.61*	.70**	NA	NA
		9 months N=12		
.42	.72**	.78**	.76**	.78**
		12 months N=19		
.78***	.56*	.36	.50*	.74***
		15 months N=19		
.67**	0	.12	.66**	.74***
		18 months N=19		
.54*	NA	NA	.78***	.48*

*p .05
**p .01
***p .001

Table 9.3. Correlations of language scores with MDI and PDI Adjusted Scores

	MDI	PDI
6 months N=16	.82***	.29
9 months N=12	.73**	.86***
12 months N=19	.66**	.30
15 months N=19	.66**	.56*
18 months N=19	.69**	.78***

*p .05
**p .01
***p .001

tions, imitation-comprehension, and vocalization-social; at 12 months, eye-hand coordination, manipulation, imitation-comprehension, and vocalization-social; at 15 months, eye-hand coordination, imitation-comprehension, and vocalization-social; and at 18 months, eye-hand coordination, imitation-comprehension, and vocalization-social. It is interesting to note that eye-hand coordination is strongly correlated with language development at all ages. However, the intermediate age levels show an increasing trend of correlation to the later developmental scales. Highest correlations of the imitation-comprehension scale were at 9 and 18 months; and for the vocalization-social scale at 9, 12, and 15 months.

The language scores also correlated significantly with the total Bayley MDI scores (range .66 to .82) and with the Bayley PDI scores (range .29 to .86), as shown in Table 9.3. Correlations were more consistent for the Mental Development Scale than they were for the Motor Development Scale.

The Binet mental age at $2\frac{1}{2}$ also correlated significantly with the Bayley MDI scores (range .62 to .79) and less significantly with PDI scores (.003 to .75). MDI scores were related across the board; PDI scores at 9, 15, and 18 months. These are shown in Table 9.4.

Table 9.4. Correlation of Binet mental age in months with Bayley MDI and PDI adjusted scores

	MDI	PDI
6 months N=16	.62**	.003
9 months N=12	.79**	.75**
12 months N=19	.71***	.29
15 months N=19	.67**	.63**
18 months N=19	.71***	.75**

*p .05
**p .01
***p .001

Table 9.5. Correlation of Bayley MDI and PDI adjusted scores at each age

Age in Months	6	9	12	15	18
			MDI		
6		.60*	.35	.59*	.60*
9			.80**	.85***	.83***
12				.87***	.86***
15					.90***
			PDI		
6		.21	.31	.18	.31
9			.81**	.79**	.84***
12				.59**	.57**
15					.84***

*p .05
**p .01
***p .001

The Bayley measures intercorrelated significantly with each other at each age, shown in Table 9.5. MDI intercorrelations ranged from .35 to .90; PDI intercorrelations from .18 to .84. The Kohen-Raz subscales correlated with Bayley MDIs from .51 to .93 where the scales were most applicable; and with PDIs from −.24 to .79 where the scales were most applicable, shown in Table 9.6. Eye-hand sub-

Table 9.6. Correlations of Kohen-Raz subscales of the Bayley with MDI and PDI adjusted scores at each age level

	Kohen-Raz Subscales				
	Eye–Hand	Manipulation	Object Relations	Imitation–Comprehension	Vocalization–Social
			6 months N=16		
MDI	.77***	.51*	.67**	0	.55*
PDI	.21	−.05	.22	0	−.24
			9 months N=12		
MDI	.66*	.74**	.85***	.85***	.83***
PDI	.71**	.67*	.76**	.78**	.76**
			12 months N=19		
MDI	.92***	.81***	.67**	.89***	.81***
PDI	.61**	.59**	.23	.64**	.51*
			15 months N=19		
MDI	.89***	0	.53*	.91***	.86***
PDI	.79***	0	.40	.63**	.58**
			18 months N=19		
MDI	.81***	0	o	.93***	.93***
PDI	.56*	0	0	.79***	.61**

*p .05
**p .01
***p .001

Table 9.7. Correlations of Kohen-Raz subscales of the Bayley with Binet mental age at $2\frac{1}{2}$ years

Eye–Hand	Manipulation	Kohen-Raz Object Relations	Imitation–Comprehension	Vocalization–Social
		6 months N=16		
.77***	.74**	.70**	NA	.72**
		9 months N=12		
.35	.79**	.78**	.87***	.84***
		12 months N=19		
.78***	.56*	.43	.58**	.84***
		15 months N =19		
.75***	0	.24	.69***	.77***
		18 months N=19		
.51*	NA	NA	.81***	.54*

*p .05
**p .01
***p .001

scales correlated well at all ages with the MDI scores. The Imitation-Comprehension and Vocalization-Social subscales correlated well past 6 months. The motor scales (PDI) were least correlated with the Kohen-Raz subscales at 6 months. These low correlations may be related to the inflation of adjusted measures (adjusted for conception age) on the motor scale at that age level.

The Kohen-Raz subscales of the Bayley correlated significantly with the Binet Mental Age at $2\frac{1}{2}$ years as well (range .24 to .84). Highest correlations were at 9 months on Imitation-Comprehension and Vocalization-Social, at 12 months on Vocalization-Social, and at 18 months on Imitation-Comprehension. These are shown in Table 9.7.

Table 9.8 shows the developmental milestones of words (15 months), sitting (11 months), crawling (11 months), walking (16 months), and sentences of 2 words (between 17 months and three years).

Objectal and object constancy correlations with language development are presented in Table 9.9. It indicates significant correlations

Table 9.8. Milestones

	Two Words	Sitting	Crawling	Walking	Sentences
N	19	12	12	19	6 and 13
Mean	14.84	11.08	10.83	16.16	16.5 and 24–36
Standard Deviation	2.27	2.50	1.80	3.24	1.64

Table 9.9. Correlation of Décarie objectal and object constancy scales with language scores

	Objectal	Object Constancy
6 months N=16	.40	.43
12 months N=16	.73*	.67*
18 months N=17	NA	.32

p .01

at 12 months, and in the predicted direction at age 6 months. The 18 months scores suffer from the ceiling effect at that age.

DISCUSSION

The controversy continues not only about the contribution of genes versus environment to later intelligence, but as to how early one can predict cognitive outcome. There has been a recent emphasis on prediction for high risk and premature infants.

The Louisville Twin Study has emphasized the importance of genetic contribution (Wilson, 1983). However, recent studies on high risk infants have cited the importance of environmental factors in prediction of outcome in these infants (Siegel, 1982; Bee et al, 1982). An important aspect of these studies is the general predictability and reliability and/or validity of infant tests as predictors of later outcome.

Ulvund (1984) in his reflections on the nature of intelligence has suggested that first of all there are two aspects of intelligence with which we are dealing: the continuity-discontinuity of developmental functions and the stability-instability in individual differences. The low correlations between infant-test results and later intelligence he indicates may represent the instability of individual differences. He further wonders whether our interest in infant test prediction should be in contemporary validity since there is discontinuity in development. Prediction, moreover, improves when specific abilities are addressed, rather than global measures.

The results of the Kohen-Raz subscales (1967) correlations with language measures and developmental test measures are highly comparable to those of Siegel (1981). The correlations were high and significant. The language scores correlated significantly with the total Bayley scores, and the Binet mental age at two and a half also correlated significantly with the Bayley MDI and PDI. The Bayley measures intercorrelated significantly with each other at each age tested, as did most of the Kohen-Raz subscales with the total Bayleys at each age tested. The Kohen-Raz subscales of the Bayley correlated highly with the Binet Mental Age at two and a half years also. The correlations of the Object Constancy and Objectal Relations scales with language development were significant only at the 12 month level, although the other ages were in the predicted direction.

Bee et al. (1982) did not find that the infant tests were predictive of later language or intellectual outcome until age two and suggests that the difference in his findings from the Siegel study (1982) may be due to the high number of premature infants in Siegel's sample with the suggestion that these tests may predict better for lower functioning infants. However, his measures were total Bayley and Binet scores. Again, it may be that when specific abilities are studied that these may better predict later outcome.

The Kohen-Raz scales (1967) that correlated significantly with language development were those of eye-hand coordination and conceptual ability at 6 months; eye-hand coordination, manipulation, imitation/comprehension and vocalization/social for 12 months; and eye-hand coordination, imitation/comprehension and vocalization/social for 18 months. This finding confirms those that Siegel (1981) found in her study using Bayley and Reynall scales of language development. She notes: "A maturational delay manifests itself in whatever behavior is predominant at that developmental stage, and those delays are significant in terms of forecasting later delays in more complex behavior" (Siegel, 1981:555).

Different patterns of behavior are predominant at different ages, and are related precursors of later more complex behavior and development. These findings are of interest because differential patterns of the Kohen-Raz scales of the Bayley were correlated with later more complex development, both language and cognitive. It is a different pattern at each age measured, furthermore, that correlates with language development at two and a half years.

The pattern that Siegel (1981) noted was that perceptual-motor items tended to be predictive early, the object relations and similar items tended to be predictive later on, and the language-related items (imitation-comprehension and vocalization-social) became predictive at 12 and 18 months. This pattern was generally replicated by our findings.

These findings seems to suggest that different measures at different ages are predictive of later more complex behaviors (and indeed, they are what can be measured at these early ages). At early ages, simple behaviors of a perceptual motor nature (and making interesting things happen) are those that seem to be precursors of later language and cognitive development. At later ages, more adaptive, imitative, and social skills are related. There is a genetic and maturational shift in the patterns of skills with developmental age. Wilson refers to these patterns as "emergent capabilities" (Wilson, 1983: 314). The plasticity of early development gives way to developmental and directional processes that are highly directed.

We have noted the pattern of shift from motor and perceptual to objectal and imitative functions to vocalization and social-communicative skills. There is emerging theory and evidence (Caron and Caron, 1981; Caron, Caron, and Glass, 1983: 184) that the precursors of language are based on earlier experience and abilities to form relationship concepts and to understand categories. We early referred in a previous chapter to the high relationship between prehension and motor skills to the development of the object concept and categorical thinking. In addition, there seems to be increasing evidence that the gestural imitation stage (Siegel, 1981; Acredolo and Goodwyn, 1985) is an important precursor to language, highly related to the motor skills that are its precursor.

It is this movement from action to language (Sanders-Woudstra, 1983) that may well be hampered in low birth weight and premature infants, and thus indeed there is an important early relationship between these measures and later outcome. Lewis and Bendersky (1989) in studying preterm infants with such medical complications as interventricular hemorrhage found that they performed significantly more poorly on measures of cognitive and motor development and language ability was correlated with other medical complications.

Table 9.8 herein indicates delays in such motor milestones as sitting, crawling, and walking, compared with Sugar's sample (Sugar, 1982) First words are at about the same level of his premature sample in our group. However, when first sentences are reviewed there is a distinct discrepancy between the higher birth weight children (Mean about 16.5 months) and the low birth weight cohorts (between 24 months and 3 years as estimated from Binet responses), and all of our sample are relatively delayed as compared with phrases of three words for his sample.

It is also of interest to note the continued relationship of objectal and object constancy measures to language development (as well as to the motor and mental measures and birth weight reported in previous chapters). The development of the object preceded mental and motor development and is highly related to cognitive level. Its progress may well be based on the motor skills required to elicit attachment, just as motor skills are important for the development of knowledge of the object and subsequent classification skills.

REFERENCES

Accredolo, L. P., and Goodwyn, S. W. 1985. Symbolic gesturing in language development. *Human Development*, 28, No., 40–49.

Bee, H. L., Barnard, K. E., Eyres, S. J., Gray, C. A., Hammond, M. A., Spietz, A. L., Snyder, C., and Clark, B. 1982. Prediction of IQ and language skill from perinatal status, child performance, family characteristics, and mother-infant interaction. *Child Development*, 53, 1134–1156.

Caron, A. J., and Caron, R. F. 1981. Chapter 12. Processing of relational information as an index of infant risk. In S. L. Friedman and M. Sigman (Eds.) *Preterm birth and psychological development*. New York: Academic Press.

Caron, A. J., Caron, R. F., and Glass, P. 1983. Chapter 9. Responsiveness to relational information as a measure of cognitive functioning in nonsuspect infants. In T. F. Field and A. Sostok (Eds.) *Infants born at risk*. New York: Grune and Stratton.

Lewis, M., and Bendersky, M. 1989. Cognitive and Motor Differences Among Low Birth Weight Infants: Impact of Intraventricular Hemorrhage, Medical Risk, and Social Class. *Pediatrics*, 83 (2), 187–192.

Siegel, L. S. 1979. Infant perceptual, cognitive, and motor behaviours as predictors of subsequent cognitive and language development. *Canadian Journal of Psychology/Review of Canadian Psychology*, 33 (4), 382–394.

Siegel, L. S. 1981. Infant tests as predictors of cognitive and language development at two years. *Child Development*, 52, 545–557.

Siegel, L. S., Saigal, S., Rosenbaum, P., Morton, R. A., Young, A., Berembaum, S., and Stoskopf, B. 1982. Predictors of development in preterm and full-term infants: A model for detecting the at risk child. *Journal of Pediatric Psychology*, 7, No. 2, 135–148.

Sugar, M. 1982. Chapter 1. Developmental Milestones in Prematures. In *The Premature in Context*. New York: SP Medical and Scientific Books.

Ulvund, S. E. 1984. Predictive validity of assessments of early cognitive competence in light of some current issues in developmental psychology. *Human Development*, 27, No. 2, 76–83.

Wilson, R. S. 1983. The Louisville Twin Study: Developmental Synchronies in Behavior. *Child Development*, 54, 298–316.

CHAPTER 10

School Days

We have demonstrated good "catch up" effect in our group of multiple birth children by 2 to 3 years of age, with outcome closer to their socioeconomic level. The literature on low birth weight children has disagreed on whether this type of "catch up" effect carries on into school days. Some have opted for the more optimistic conclusion that birth weight and prematurity effects are outgrown (Benton, 1940).

Prematurity and low birth weight have been generally recognized as main variables in affecting delay among low birth weight, preterm singleton infants during the first two years of life (Davies and Stewart, 1975; Hunt and Rhodes, 1977; Wiener, 1962). Cohen, Parmalee, Sigman, and Beckwith (1988) have concluded that language and symbolic deficits dating from the second year of life have implications for later learning difficulties. There is some disagreement as to whether the main effect is birth weight, or perinatal neurological deficits associated with birth weight that influence developmental level (Harper and Wiener, 1965; Braine, Helmer, Worthis, and Freedman, 1966). Other scientists have suggested that these effects persist into school years in the form of learning disability (Davies and Stewart, 1975; Rubin, Rosenblatt, and Balow, 1973; Stewart and Reynolds, 1974; Wiener, 1962; Caputo, Goldstein, and Taub, 1979; and Caputo, Goldstein, and Taub, 1981).

The longitudinal data on this sample of multiple birth children has demonstrated that on the average this group of children do catch up by two years of age and that birth weight effects diminish by three years of age. However, the later intellectual test data at seven and nine years of age reveals that by school age some of the children are being targeted as having school problems.

RESULTS

Table 10.1 presents the longitudinal developmental mental scores on the Bayley Infant Scale, Stanford Binet, Form L-M Intelligence test.

Table 10.1. Developmental scores of multiple birth children

	Adjusted Scores Bayley MDI Scores					Birth Scores Binet IQs				
Age	3	6	9	12	15	18	24	30	36	60
N	16	16	12	19	19	19	19	19	19	19
Mean	115	115	98	100	106	109	116	126	129	127
S.D.	16.1	17.6	18.9	18.3	23.0	22.2	22.2	22.0	13.8	18.0

Adjusted measures for conception age through three years of age reveal functioning close to the standardization average by 9 months of age. They are somewhat above that at 3 and 6 months of age, possibly due to inflation as a result of the correction. These corrections were not done past 3 years of age. By 3 years of age, the scores are well above average. The children retain this above average functioning through 5 years of age. However, with the change to the Wechsler Intelligence Scale for Children, Revised, scores diminish to the upper limit of the average range of intelligence. (Please refer to Table 10.2.) You will note some discrepancy in the number of subjects for the Wechsler data. All nineteen subjects were seen at age 7; one cohort was seen at age 8. At age 9, fourteen of the original subjects were seen, and a new set of identical triplet girls were added to the sample. The followup data are for one cohort at age 12. The data are remarkably stable on the Wechsler Scale for these ages, 7, 8, 9, and the followup measure at age 12.

An examination of the individual subtest scores of the Wechsler Intelligence Scale for Children, Revised in Table 10.3 for age 7 shows no significant differences in subtest score for all children combined. This consistency of performance continues at age 9, shown in Table 10.5. There were, however, five children in four families that were identified as having learning problems and for whom special classes

Table 10.2. Wechsler Intelligence Scale for children, revised IQs

Age	7 years	8 years	9 years	12 years
N	19	*	17	*
VIQ	115	107	110	110
Range	97–147	103–109	90–135	105–113
S.D.	15.9	2.6	12.4	3.4
PIQ	109	106	108	97
Range	92–131	85–115	91–147	74–105
S.D.	11.8	12.2	13.6	15.2
Full IQ	114	107	110	104
Range	96–131	95–112	89–144	92–115
S.D.	15.4	6.7	13.8	8.9

*One cohort.

Table 10.3. Average subtest scores of the Wechsler Intelligence Scale, revised, age seven

	Verbal Scale				
	Information	Similarities	Arithmetic	Vocabulary	Comprehension
Mean	12.1	13.2	11.1	13.2	12.3
S.D.	2.7	2.9	3.0	3.5	2.9
	Performance Scale				
	Picture Completion	Picture Arrangement	Block Designs	Object Assembly	Coding
Mean	10.5	12.2	11.8	10.8	12.2
S.D.	2.6	1.9	2.8	2.3	2.5

or tutoring was recommended. Three of these children came from cohorts where there were high risk factors, reported in Table 1.1

One of these cohorts constitutes the one studied at age 8 and followed up at age 12. If one looks at the individual subtests (see Tables 10.4 and 10.6), one can see that at age 8, the Arithmetic score is below the level of the other verbal subtests. By age twelve, this differential is not maintained for this cohort, but two other subtests

Table 10.4. Average subtest scores of the Wechsler Intelligence Scale, revised, age eight

	Verbal Scale				
	Information	Similarities	Arithmetic	Vocabulary	Comprehension
Mean	13.2	9.8	8.8	12.8	11.6
S.D.	.9	1.3	1.1	1.6	.6
	Performance Scale				
	Picture Completion	Picture Arrangement	Block Designs	Object Assembly	Coding
Mean	10.4	10.2	10.2	9.2	14.6
S.D.	1.7	3.1	2.1	1.8	2.2

Table 10.5. Average subtest scores of the Wechsler Intelligence Scale, revised, age nine

	Verbal Scale				
	Information	Similarities	Arithmetic	Vocabulary	Comprehension
Mean	10.8	12.8	10.8	12.4	12.0
S.D.	2.3	2.8	2.3	2.4	2.9
	Performance Scale				
	Picture Completion	Picture Arrangement	Block Designs	Object Assembly	Coding
Mean	9.9	11.2	11.7	10.9	12.5
S.D.	2.5	3.6	2.6	2.6	2.5

Table 10.6. Average subtest scores of the Wechsler Intelligence Scale, revised, age twelve

	Verbal Scale				
	Information	Similarities	Arithmetic	Vocabulary	Comprehension
Mean	11.0	12.2	10.2	Not given	13.4
S.D.	2.1	1.3	1.1		1.3
	Performance Scale				
	Picture Completion	Picture Arrangement	Block Designs	Object Assembly	Coding
Mean	8.6	9.4	8.6	Not given	12.0
S.D.	2.1	1.7	2.3		4.5

show decrement, Picture Completion and Block Designs. It must be noted that these findings are on the average, and one targeted child contributes to these decrements heavily.

The five targeted learning difficulty children were compared with those not identified as having learning problems on the WISC-R subtests, and the difference between the two groups studied by Chi-Square, at ages 7 and 9.

We compared each child on each of his subtests with the average of his own subtests on the Verbal and Performance Scales respectively. An indicator of weakness on a subtest was defined by a score that was lower than twice the standard error of measurement for that subtest. For Table 10.7, where the 7 year old scores are used, the standard error of measurement used was that for 7½ year olds (Table 10, WISC-R Manual). For Table 10.8, where the 9 year old scores are studied, the standard error of measurement used was that for 10½ year olds (see Table 10, WISC-R Manual).

For age 7, the targeted children all obtained such weakness indicators as compared with 7 of the 14 nontargeted children. The Chi-Square was 5.5, significant at the .02 level of confidence. Subtest scores most often lower than twice the standard error of measurement were the Picture Completion and the Arithmetic subtests of the WISC-

Table 10.7. Comparison of targeted learning problem children with non-targeted children on the Wechsler subtest scales, at seven

	Indicators Present	Indicators Absent
Targeted Children	5	0
Non-Targeted	7	7
Degrees of Freedom	1	
Chi-Square	5.5	
Level of Confidence	.02	

Table 10.8. Comparison of targeted learning problem children with non-targeted children on the Wechsler subtest scales, at nine

	Indicators Present	Indicators Absent
Targeted Children	2	2
Non-Targeted	1	13
Degrees of Freedom	1	
Chi-Square	12.0	
Level of Confidence	.01	

R. This suggests some combination of perceptual and numerical abstract reasoning impairments, which may relate highly to their school difficulties.

At age 9, the number of targeted children showing subtests lower than twice the standard error of measurement were 2 out of 4 remaining in the included sample at age 9, while only 1 out of 13 nontargeted children did so. The Chi-Square for these results was 12.0, significant beyond the .01 level of confidence. The two targeted children in this sample showed their low scores on Arithmetic. As indicated above, for Tables 10.4 and 10.6 there is one targeted child contributing to low scores on Picture Completion and Block Designs. There continues to be consistency in the scores that are low, having to do with perceptual and numerical reasoning.

DISCUSSION

The longitudinal data on these multiple birth children, some of whom were preterm and of low birth weight, indicates that on the average there is "catch up" by at least two years of age, and birth weight effects diminished by two and three years of age. There has, however, been some recent concern that the age corrections (used in this study to 3 years of age), ignore high risk factors such as perinatal neurological complications and other factors related to the intrauterine crowding of multiple birth children, that may interfere with later development (Caputo, Goldstein, and Taub, 1981). The correction is viewed as equalizing premature infants with full term infants, thus ignoring other high risk factors that may later emerge.

The above average adjusted mental scores at 3 months and 6 months may reflect a combination of overcorrection of scores for prematurity, or artifacts in the scales at those ages, and/or advantage of increased extrauterine experiences associated with prematurity, which diminish during the second half of the first year. The increases in scores past two years may reflect the increased socialization experiences of their high socioeconomic status and stimulation from multiple siblings. There is growing evidence from the longitudinal studies on prediction for outcome of high risk infants that the social and caregiver interaction effects on later outcome are as significant as other factors in prediction (Cohen and Parmalee, 1983).

However, the school age scores show that on the average there is a drop in score from the preschool measures, and four families have identified learning problem children. Not all of these children were of low birthweight. The data suggest that either high risk factors are surfacing in later school years, or the change in test measure accounts entirely for the drop in score close to one standard deviation. The latter is highly unlikely. The WISC-R manual reports highly similar IQs at ages 6 and 9½ for their standardization sample. The five targeted learning problem children moreover, all had some subtest scores lower than twice the standard error of measurement for their age group, in comparison with those children not so targeted. This is similar to Hunt's (1981) findings that children targeted with problems tended to persist in having those problems between ages 4–6 to 8 years of age. Interestingly enough, the differences were greater for performance scores. This is similar to our findings that the subtests most vulnerable for the mentioned children were Picture Completion and Arithmetic. Caputo et al. (1981) found that the subtests on which the prematures had most difficulty were Block Design, Object Assembly, and Picture Completion for Performance scale; and Arithmetic, for the Verbal scale. Lefebvre, Bard, Veilleuz, and Martel (1988) found a verbal score substantially lower than the performance score for children below 1000 grams. Some of these differences in findings may relate to sample differences in socioeconomic status. Lloyd, Wheldall, and Perks (1988) have pointed out that the size of differences between the IQs of their low birth weight and control children was similar to that of those seen between children with the same birthweight but from different social classes.

A comparison of our developmental scores at 5, 7, and 9 with those in the relevant literature shows that the absolute level of our scores is somewhat higher than those reported. Cohen and Parmalee (1983) report an average Binet IQ of 104.6 for their English speaking children. Caputo et al. report an average Verbal IQ for their total sample of 104.0, 101.7 for the Performance IQ, and 103.5 for their Full Scale IQ. These scores are higher than for their low birth weight children, but their higher birth weight children's scores are more comparable to our overall average (Verbal IQ 106.0, Performance IQ 112.4, and Full Scale IQ 110.0).

McCall et al. (1973) report an overall average IQ for the multiple births in the Fels project of 102. They reported at that time that only six of their 30 multiple births had an average IQ above the Fels mean (approximately 117 on the Binet at age 10), and 14 had averages lower than 1 standard deviation below the Fels mean. Note that our final mean Full IQ score was on the average (110). Six of our sample had IQs above their own average, and 11 below from those tested at age 9.

While there seems to be some diminishing of the scores between 5 and 7, our group tends to demonstrate caregiver and socioeconomic effect. The most recent literature continues to demonstrate that the early measures on premature high risk infants show greatest deficits in motor scores (Ross, 1985). Ross (1985) wonders whether these perceptual-motor and related deficits will manifest themselves later in other cognitive, motor, and behavioral areas as the child matures. In our sample, the test scores are on the average higher than reported elsewhere in the literature. However, there are some high risk effects also emerging in the form of reported learning problems, which occurred in high as well as low birthweight multiples. These were identified quickly with our regular testing schedules, and the children's needs for remediation were addressed quickly. In our families, coming as they are from middle class families, other emotional and social amenities have been available to the children to enhance their cognitive and emotional development. Emotional development will be reported upon in the next chapter.

REFERENCES

Bayley, N. 1969. *Manual for the Bayley Scales of Infant Development.* New York: The Psychological Corporation.

Benton, A. 1940. Mental development of prematurely born children. *American Journal of Orthopsychiatry.* 10, 719–746.

Braine, M. D. S., Helmer, C. B., Worthis, H., and Freedman, A. M. 1966. Factors associated with impairment of the early development of prematures. *Monographs of the Society for Research in Child Development*, 31, 4.

Caputo, D. V., Goldstein, K. M., and Taub, H. B. 1979. Chapter 11. The development of prematurely born children through middle childhood. In T. M. Field, A. M. Sostek, S. Goldberg and H. H. Shuman (Eds.) *Infants born at risk.* New York: SP Medical and Scientific Books.

Caputo, D. V., Goldstein, K. M., and Taub, H. B. 1981. Chapter 20. Neonatal compromise and later psychological development. In S. L. Friedman and M. Sigman (Eds.) *Preterm birth and psychological development*. New York: Academic Press.

Cohen, S. E., and Parmalee, A. H. 1983. Prediction of five-year Stanford Binet scores in preterm infants. *Child Development*. 54, 1242–1253.

Cohen, S. E., Parmalee, A. H., Sigman, M., and Beckwith, L. 1988. Antecedents of School Problems in Children Born Preterm. *Journal of Pediatrics*. 13 (4), 493–508.

Davies, P, and Stewart, A. L. 1975. Low birth-weight infants: Neurological sequelae and later intelligence. *British Medical Bulletin*. 31, 85–91.

Harper, P. A., and Wiener, G. 1965. Sequelae of low birth weight. *Annual Review of Medicine*. 16, 405–420.

Hunt, J. V. 1981. Chapter 19. Predicting intellectual disorders in childhood for preterm infants with birthweights below 1501 gm. In S. L. Friedman and M. Sigman (Eds.) *Preterm birth and psychological development*. New York: Academic Press.

Hunt, J. V., and Rhodes, L. 1977. Mental development of pre-term infants during the first year. *Child Development*. 48, 204–210.

Lefebvre, F., Bard, H., Veilleuz, A., and Martel, C. 1988. Outcome at school age of children with birthweights of 1000 grams or less. *Developmental Medicine and Child Neurology*. 30 (2), 170–181.

Lloyd, B. W., Wheldall, K., and Perks, D. 1988. Controlled study of intelligence and school performance of very low birthweight children from a defined geographical area. *Developmental Medicine and Child Neurology*. 30 (1), 36–43.

McCall, R. B., Appelbaum, M. I., and Hogarty, D. S. 1973. Developmental changes in mental performance. *Monographs of the Society for Research in Child Development*. 38, No. 3.

Ross, G. 1985. Use of the Bayley Scales to Characterize Abilities of Premature Infants. *Child Development*. 56, 835–842.

Rubin, A., Rosenblatt, C., and Balow, B. 1973. Psychological and educational sequelae of prematurity. *Pediatrics*. 52: 352–363.

Stewart, A., and Reynolds, . 1974. Improved prognosis for infants of very low birth weight. *Pediatrics*. 54, 6, 724–735.

Terman, D. M., and Merrill, M. A. 1973. *Stanford-Binet Intelligence Scale*. Boston: Houghton Mifflin Company.

Wechsler, D. 1974. *Wechsler Intelligence Scale for Children, Revised*. New York: The Psychological Corporation.

Wiener, G. 1962. Psychological correlates of premature birth: A review. *Journal of Nervous and Mental Diseases*. 134, 129–144.

CHAPTER 11

Personality Development

There has been considerable interest in the multiple birth status of twins as to the effect of twin status, and particularly identical versus fraternal status of twinship, on personality development. There has been less opportunity to study these effects on the personality development of multiples beyond twins. Twin reports are suggestive that twin status does have some influence on personality development (Bank & Kahn, 1982; Ainslee, 1985). Ainslee (1985) has identified several stress points in the life of twins for the development of identity. The initial stress point is the first six months of life, with the vicissitudes of the mother-infant dyad in view of the often high risk status of the infant and the exhaustion of caring for more than one infant at a time. The second is the rapprochement phase between 18 and 24 months, when there are stresses of separation-individuation, caused both by depletion from the previous phase, and excessive intertwin identification, i.e. using the twin as a transitional object. The third stress point is at adolescence, when identity formation is reworked.

In this chapter, we will examine whether multiple birth cohorts beyond twins are similar or dissimilar in their object representations and in their methods of coping with the phase stresses of the ages studied, five, seven, eight, nine, and a followup for one cohort at age twelve. We are interested in whether they show these same stresses in identity formation.

The method that we will use to study identity formation is by tracing the object representation through these various ages. Winnicott (1975) traces the development of the object into the following stages: (1) Subject relates to the object; (2) the object is found instead of placed by the subject in the world; (3) Subject destroys the object; (4) Object survives destruction; and (5) Subject can use the object. Further to quote: "the paradox and the acceptance of the paradox: the baby creates the object, but the object was there waiting to be created and to become a cathected object" (Winnicott, 1975).

The general method we will use for tracing the use of the object will be that of the Rorschach ink blot test, given to all subjects at five and later. A Rorschach assumption (Exner & Weiner, 1983) is that the human movement (M) represents for the child a recreation of his object world. This develops in transition between the ages of approximately five and seven, when normatively between .8 and 1.7 M responses are given, and 1.6 and 1.9 human responses (Exner & Weiner, 1983). The precursors to this development are his quasi-human responses, such as animals in some type of human movement, monsters and witches, and part-body human percepts.

Through the Rorschach object responses depicted in the ink blot records, we should be able to make some inferences as to the level of development towards the ability to use the object. Another way of phrasing this is that with the ability to use the object a stronger sense of identity and self has emerged. We may ask whether the child is at the stage of finding the object; destroying the object; or using the object, to bind the impulses generated by the stimulating ink blots and their own inner psychic status.

PROCEDURES

Beginning at the age of five in this longitudinal study, the children were administered the Rorschach Ink Blot test and Human Figure drawing test, following the intelligence test for the appropriate age. The administrations occurred within four weeks of their birthdays. Except for one family, these occurred in their own home. One family came to the clinic for the test series, and the examination was done in sequence while the other children were visiting with mother in the waiting room or close by. The same examiner or examiners tested the children and was/were well known to the families.

The Rorschach ink blot test was scored by the Exner Comprehensive scoring system, and compared with Exner norms (Exner & Weiner, 1983). In addition, all human and quasi-human responses were scored and evaluated with two scales: the Pruitt and Spilka scale (Pruitt & Spilka, 1964), and the Blatt Object Representations Scale (Blatt, 1976). The Pruitt and Spilka scale scores were correlated with human figure drawings results as scored by the Harris system (1963) and with Stanford Binet, Form L-M intelligence test IQs (Terman & Merrill, 1973), and Wechsler Intelligence Scale for Children,

Revised IQs (Wechsler, 1974. The results of the Blatt scale will be discussed in the clinical section of the chapter. A more detailed description of the two object representational scales is given in Chapter 4 above.

RESULTS

The comparison of the Rorschach scores with Exner norms for age 5 (see Table 11.1) indicate significant differences from the norms at the .05 level of confidence or lower in the following scoring categories: R, D, F+%, FM, CF, C, Affective ratio, P, and Zf, all in a lower direction than the norms. When the .01 level of confidence is accepted, the scores that remain are R, FM, CF, C, Affective Ratio, P, Zf, and (2)/R or egocentricity index. The only score that was higher than the norms, at the .05 level of confidence, was the FC response. It should be noted that these differences were small. For example, R averaged 12.32 as compared with Exner norms of 15.2 for five year olds. One record had 6 responses, lower than the 10 responses recommended for statistical comparison with Exner norms. However, the combined results suggest more constriction and control than his normative sample, combined with a slightly lower accuracy level and conventionality.

This same comparison with Exner norms was made for age 7 (see Table 11.2). Scores that show a difference in a lower direction at the .05 level of confidence are Dd, F+%, X+%, C, and A%. Scores lower than Exner norms at the .01 level of confidence are FM, Affective Ratio, Zf, and (2)/R or the egocentricity index. Scores higher than Exner norms at the .05 level of confidence are D and FC, and m at the .01 level of confidence. These findings are remarkably consistent with the 5 year results, and with a higher response rate of 20.63 as compared with 18.3 for the Exner sample. The comparison with Exner ratios at this age level is more than justified. The sample continues to demonstrate more personality constriction; a lower level of conventionality, and a more practical, less wholistic or organizational approach to their environment. There seems to be a more socialized orientation, with less impulsivity, and more socialization anxiety (FC,m), than the Exner normative sample.

This same comparison for age 9 is reported in Table 11.3 for a sample that includes one different cohort. As indicated above in Chapter 10, one of the original cohorts was tested at age 8 instead of 9, and a set of identical triplet girls is added to the sample at age

Table 11.1. Rorschach scoring categories (age 5, N = 19)

	R	W	D	Dd	F+%	X+%	M	Fm	m	FC	CF
Mean	12.32	8.21	3.84	.21	73.11	73	.68	.79	.21	1.32	.84
SD	2.40	1.72	3.13	.54	16.23	17.64	.95	1.13	.42	1.38	1.07
Exner	15.2	9.2	5.6	.4	.83	.81	.8	2.8	.1	.5	1.9
t	3.39	1.84	2.30	1.43	2.58	1.92	.53	6.86	.52	2.42	4.12
p	.01	NS	.05	NS	.05	NS	NS	.01	NS	.05	.01

	C	Aff/R	C'	Y	T	V	A%	P	Zf	L	H	(2)/R
Mean	.11	.43	.68	1.47	0	.11	47.37	2.68	9	1.87	.95	.16
SD	.46	.15	1.25	2.52	0	.32	23.35	1.49	1.53	2.32	1.39	.17
Exner	.9	1.07	.3	.5	.8	0	.54	3.8	10.6	1.14	1.6	.61
t	5.98	6.4	.41	1.64	.8	.73	1.21	3.11	3.17	1.10	.75	10.98
p	.01	.01	NS	NS	NS	NS	NS	.01	.01	NS	NS	.01

Table 11.2. Rorschach scoring categories (age 7, N = 19)

	R	W	D	Dd	F + %	X + %	M	FM	m	FC	CF
Mean	20.63	6.32	8.63	.42	73	75	2.05	1.32	1.16	2.26	.58
SD	23.09	1.89	4.62	.69	24.89	17.42	1.90	1.42	1.64	2.10	1.02
Exner	18.3	9.1	7.60	1.6	86	84	1.70	3.6	.3	1.20	2.6
t	.43	1.66	2.34	2.24	2.21	2.19	.78	6.33	5.73	2.16	7.77
p	NS	NS	.05	.05	.05	.05	NS	.01	.01	.05	.01

	C	Aff/R	C'	Y	T	V	A%	P	Zf	L	H	(2)/R
Mean	.26	.47	1.63	.47	.89	.21	44	4.16	8.26	1.68	4.26	.26
SD	.73	.27	3.47	.70	2.51	.54	14.04	1.46	2.26	2.86	2.00	.13
Exner	.6	.84	.5	.5	.8	.1	51	4.0	10.6	.91	4.1	.61
t	2.00	6.17	1.38	.19	.15	1.62	2.11	.43	4.03	1.15	.31	11.67
p	.05	.01	NS	NS	NS	NS	.05	NS	.01	NS	NS	.01

Table 11.3. Rorschach scoring categories (age 9, N = 17)

	R	W	D	Dd	F+%	X+%	M	FM	m	FC	CF
Mean	21.12	6.76	12.06	2.29	65	70	2.18	1.00	.35	2.88	0
SD	11.19	4.84	9.69	3.53	16.09	14.90	2.56	1.27	.61	3.22	0
Exner	20.3	9.8	7.6	1.6	86	84	1.7	3.6	.3	1.2	2.6
t	.29	2.45	1.84	.78	5.22	3.75	.75	7.43	.45	2.07	23.64
p	NS	.05	NS	NS	.01	.01	NS	.01	NS	.05	.01

	C	Aff/R	C′	Y	T	V	A%	P	Zf	L	H	(2)/R
Mean	.06	.47	.88	.88	.24	.18	51	4.35	8.41	2.62	5.59	.30
SD	.24	.15	1.17	2.64	.44	.53	13.44	1.27	5.39	1.95	3.54	.19
Exner	.60	.84	.5	.5	.8	.01	51	4.0	10.6	.91	4.1	.61
t	9.00	9.25	1.31	.58	4.67	1.38	0	1.00	1.60	3.49	1.64	5.2
p	.01	.01	NS	NS	.01	NS	NS	NS	NS	.01	NS	.01

Table 11.4. Correlations of object scores with Human Figure Drawing scores and Stanford Binet, Form L-M IQs (age 5, N = 19)

	Object Scores	Human Figure Drawing Scores	Stanford Binet Form L-M IQs
Object Scores		−.20, p NS	−.16, p NS
Mean	33.84		
SD	24.44		
Human Figure Drawing Scores			.46, p .05
Mean		88.16	
SD		11.76	
Stanford Binet, Form L-M IQs			
Mean			127.11
SD			17.95

9. For this sample, the rate of response is again slightly but not significantly higher than the Exner sample. The mean rate of response is 21.12 as compared with 20.3 for the normative sample. Scores that are lower than the Exner sample at the .05 level are for W, and at the .01 level of confidence, they are F+%, X+%, FM, CF, C, Affective Ratio, T, and (2)/R or egocentricity index. Higher scores are for FC (.05 level) and Lambda (.01 level). The findings continue to suggest a less wholistic and less conventional approach, with more socialization controls, less impulsivity, and more constriction.

To pursue our interest in the object representations and their reflection of identity devlopment in our sample, we utilized the Pruitt and Spilka scale (1964). This scale gives weighted scores for all percepts from humans in movement with sex specified in present temporal context (18) to animals in human like action(1). The scale is discussed in more detail in Chapter 4. At age 5, there was a wide range of variability in the content of our records from 0 presence of human or quasi-human content to a weighted score of 83 for one subject. The mean score was 33.84 and the standard deviation was 24.44. (See Table 11.4) When these scores are correlated with the scores on the Human Figure Drawings and with the Stanford Binet, Form L-M IQs, there is no relationship. It had been expected that there might be a relationship to the human figure drawings, since these have often been described as representing the self or object representation of the individual who executes the drawing. However, it is also a matter of record (Harris, 1963) that the figure drawing scores are highly correlated with intelligence. There was a slight trend for the object scale measure to be negatively related to the human

Table 11.5. Correlations of object scores with Human Figure Drawing Scores and Wechsler Intelligence Scale IQs (age 7, N = 19)

	Object Scores	Human Figure Drawing Scores	Wechsler Intelligence Scale, Revised
Object Scores		.08, p NS	.21, p NS
Mean	50.26		
SD	31.76		
Human Figure Drawing Scores			.79, p .001
Mean		98.58	
SD		14.95	
Wechsler Intelligence Scale, Revised			
Mean			113.32
SD			14.58

figure drawings and to the Binet IQs, suggesting that the Pruitt and Spilka object scale is measuring something entirely different. On the other hand, the human figure drawing scores and the IQ measures are significantly correlated at the .05 level of confidence.

These findings continue to be replicated at ages 7 and 9 (see Tables 11.5 and 11.6). There is no relationship between the object scores and the human figure drawing scores and IQs, but there is a relationship between the human figure drawing scores and the IQs (significant at the .001 level of confidence at age 7 and at the .10 level of confidence at age 9). As the weighted score measure of object representation represented by the Pruitt and Spilka scale was not contributing to our understanding of the object representations of our subjects, we have turned to a more clinical approach to study the self development of our sample. We do have available for this ex-

Table 11.6. Correlations of object scores with Human Figure Drawing Scores and Wechsler Intelligence Scale IQs (age 9, N = 17)

	Object Scores	Human Figure Drawing Scores	Wechsler Intelligence Scale, Revised
Object Scores		.22, NS	.20, NS
Mean	58.59		
SD	29.64		
Human Figure Drawing Scores			.43, p .10
Mean		96.65	
SD		15.03	
Wechsler Intelligence Scale, Revised			
Mean			110.12
SD			13.77

amination the Blatt Object Representation Scale, again described in more detail in Chapter 4.

DISCUSSION

The Rorschach determinants and response numbers for this sample of multiple birth children suggested greater constriction and intellectual controls at age 5. By ages 7 and 9 the response number had increased, but was not significantly different from the Exner normative sample. There continued, however, to be more constriction in determinants, and less accuracy and less conventionality. The personality ink blot protocols were closer to both Exner and Ames norms for the number and amount of human content for all ages. Affectively across all ages this sample showed greater control and less impulsivity as a group than the Exner norms. At the earlier ages, there seemed to be a relative preoccupation with quasi-human percepts.

This preoccupation with quasi-human percepts, often of malevolent intent (monsters, Dracula, etc.) suggests that for some the level of object development was that of the destruction of the object (Winnicott, 1975), or the perception of the object as bad or not-me. However, there is in most of the records enough of the good-me or use of the object (angel, fairy godmother, girls and women, people such as two men drinking wine) to suggest the capacity to use the object for soothing and remembering for control of impulsivity. One wonders then whether the overcontrol was in the service of the ego for control of impulse and in the direction of sublimation and neutralization of aggression. It suggests some precocity in the development of social controls, possibly related to the multiple birth socialization experience, i.e. multiple siblings.

This hypothesis is supported by the gradual move of human figures toward increasing actualization in the subsequent ages studied, as detailed above. There seemed to be a movement from quasi-human figures to humans in active struggle (shooting fire) with evidence in some of the records of a move back and forth between these active and some malevolent quasi-human responses to benevolent activities, such as kissing, clapping hands, etc.

Our cohorts are different from each other, and the children within cohorts are also variable from one another, including girls from girls, and boys from boys. There did not seem to be any consistent sex differences.

Rorschach studies of monozygotic twins have generally shown greater similarity between monozygotic twins than for dizygotic twins, and our basic sample is fraternal (Basit, 1972; Hamilton, Blewitt, & Sydiaha, 1971; Rich, Greenfield, Alexander, & Sternbach, 1976). This suggests that there is not only greater genetic variability within our cohorts, but also greater environmental differential in the treatment of our children.

The two identical sibling cohorts (one set of identical twin girls studied at age seven and one set of identical triplet girls studied at age nine) that were added to the sample for comparison did show greater delay in the development of the object and seemed to be more similar to each other than to the other cohorts in the basic sample. However, these girls differed from each other in other personality features. The basic fraternal sample had a few references noted above to being stuck together, or looking like identical twins. By ages 9 and 12 these references had dropped out, and their personality protocols did not appear to show a struggle with the need to differentiate from their siblings.

The differential treatment given our sample was frequently noted in our visits to the children. The parents (usually the mother) often reported variable reactions to their children, and that they responded differently and differentially to them. Children were separated and placed in different classrooms in school. In one cohort, each year the children were given their choice as to which sibling they would be in class with that year. The children were reported to have friendships outside of the family as often as they played with their own siblings. This was particularly true of girl siblings when there was only one of them among several boy siblings. Efforts were made to treat them as individuals. Children were given different social and cultural activities according to their individual interests.

We note that Goshen-Gottstein (1980) reports that some mothers focus on similarities in their multiple-birth children; while others individualize on the basis of differences in sex, behavioral and personality characteristics. She points to the importance of these individuation tendencies in the determinants of the self-concepts of the children. It would appear that our mothers have been successful in treating their children as individuals, as our children seem to indeed be different in the personality profiles as measured in the Rorschach protocols.

The question has been raised as to whether there is a kibbutz personality, where multiple parenting is characteristic. Twenty Years

Later (1982) suggests that this is not so. The authors of this followup of kibbutz children do not find affect and attachments more moderate and diffuse. Clearly so with our multiple birth sample: the children are lively, creative, spontaneous, and different from one another, with good attachments to others as well as to each other and parental figures. At age nine, the latest year that all were studied, they were well on the way toward development of independent self concepts. Our followup cohort at age twelve are examples of the evident reworking of identity at adolescence, showing the children becoming their own persons.

CLINICAL EVALUATION

The Blatt Scale of Object Representations (1976) measures the differentiation, accuracy, level of integration, motivation, congruence of action, affective benevolence or malevolence of action, and activity level of the human or quasi-human responses on the Rorschach. While there is no quantitative score assigned to these measures, a study of the records utilizing this scale gives one an understanding of the object level of the response in a given record.

At five years of age, the human response is normatively beginning to develop. This development is preceded by a focus on animal responses, and then quasi-human and part-body human percepts. On the average, our group of 19 children gave .95 human as compared with 1.6 in the Exner group, and 1.3 in the Ames group for five year olds (Ames, Metraux, Rodell, & Walker, 1974). The main responses were quasi-humans, with a focus on monsters, witches, ghosts, dracula, batman, and more benign figures, such as fairy godmother, and angels. For the most part, responses given were only briefly described, with few details articulated. The most frequent articulation was of clothing and sex, with role sometimes implied as in witch or fairy godmother. Actions tended to be intentional, and most frequently congruent with the type of figure depicted. However, monsters were a frequent percept, and here intentionality and congruence were absent.

In general, the protocols showed a preoccupation with malevolent and fearful percepts. This seems to be consistent with the phallic phase of development and its concerns with phallic and castration level fears, and in this sense phase appropriate. However, some of the children had outgrown this preoccupation to the extent that more benign quasi-humans were given, and that more full human percepts with or without movement were there to bind the aggressive impulses rather than project and displace them. This can be inferred as a capacity to use the object for soothing. In some of the records, one could see this process in the sequence of responses. Full humans followed by phobic responses would then again be followed by human content. There seemed to be an even flow of impulse expression and the perception of the object as a form of control and internal soothing and remembering.

The level of development of the group as a whole is suggested by the noting that of the 19 records, 13 of them had some whole human form (use of the object), 4 records had human detail or quasi-human content, and only 2 records were without human or quasi-human form of any kind. However, as noted, there is considerable preoccupation at the level of destroying the object (monster, dracula, etc.) rather than at the level of use of the object. An intermediate step between the quasi-human percepts and the full human percepts are records which have pary-body parts (nose, sad or happy face) that suggest a part-body development of the object representation for soothing and neutralizing. Accompanying many of the records is a preoccupation with blackness of the blots, one child saying these are "scary," a finding for this age which Ames also reports (1974).

In examining the records for each cohort as a group, there is considerable variability between cohort members, and also variability between boys and girls. There is a considerable amount of overlap in the types of object representations between cohorts. There is, however, a trend for cohorts to be productive of object representations, or underproductive. The most productive cohort, a set of triplets, also showed the most advanced human percepts. One boy showed a clear identification with the masculine: "man with a beard" and "2 men drinking wine." Another cohort with a similar level of development demonstrates more identification with the feminine, giving people responses, including girls and women to card VII (where women are often given and this has been named the "mother" card). A more direct indicator of this level of development occurs in another well developed cohort where one percept is "a mommy and a daddy". One cohort was particularly underproductive, with a suggestion of use of intellectualization and oppositionality and overcontrol against impulses. This cohort was clearly different from the others. They had percepts close to human or quasi-human (gorilla sitting on a stick, giant with big feet); there seemed to be an identification with a powerful figure to handle the feelings of vulnerability. There thus seemed to be a wide range of development of use of the object for soothing between cohorts, and within cohorts, at this age level, with some evidence for a general age appropriateness level of phobic projection in many.

The change of object development at age 7 is striking with the full emergence of the human figure for all cohorts, even for the least productive. The number of humans and quasi humans varied from cohort to cohort. For example, cohort 1 has 14 humans, and 2 quasi humans; Cohort 2 has 6 humans, 7 quasi humans, and 2 human details; Cohort 3 has 12 humans and 3 quasi humans; Cohort 4 has 2 humans, and 9 quasi humans; and Cohort 5 has 6 humans and 5 quasi humans. No record is without some human form. We see the development of the internal capacity to use the object for soothing. Of all these percepts, 16 are "malevolent" or fearful percepts, while 52 are classified as "benevolent" This is indeed in sharp contrast to the more fearful percepts described at age 5.

As can be seen from these figures, there is some variability between cohorts, with one in particular remaining more at the level of the quasi human form of development. Examples of some of the percepts that are given by each cohort may give us some idea of how the human identity forms are acting to bind and direct impulse life, and the level of identity development of the self representation. One girl describes "two people with a bow shaking hands." Another speaks of "two people kissing each other." The activity level of these responses suggests rapprochement to form relationships that aid in meeting dependency needs, with good movement towards use of the object. In those records where this has not been fully attained, there are percepts suggesting struggle with separation and individuation issues. In some, the struggle is reflected in an active passive conflict. An active response, such as "two people on a mountain shaking hands having a fire" is followed in one record by a static human response not in movement and a fearful response, "a giant" then regression to a part body level, "a stick with two arms", followed with the recoverability of "two people sitting on two rocks, looking at each other." Then there is a final bursting through of a highly active and aggressive response: "an army shooting fire at each other." This sequence suggests a lack of comfort with inner impulses and difficulty in using the internalized object to neutralize aggression.

Another reflection of difficulty in the full internalized use of the object that seems more directly rooted in the separation individuation process are responses suggesting being stuck in the symbiotic relationship with the parental figure. In one girl, she begins with "two men pulling a girl." This anxious response is followed by "two men clapping." However, "their knees are together." One can see the sequence here of the anxious response to aggression, the rapprochement to the internalized parental surrogate for soothing, an active seeking out of the parental surrogate, in the clapping of hands. The active seeking out of the internalized object becomes clingy and inseparable and body boundaries become blurred (knees together) under the stress of the projected aggression.

In the cohort which had the fewest full human percepts, there seemed to be a closer resemblance of the records to the level of phallic-phobic preoccupations and quasi human level of the previously described 5 year Rorschach records. There seems to be a developmental progression demonstrated between these cohorts from the more overt phallic phobic struggle to a more overt active passive struggle, and then the separation individuation references described above. It is interesting to note that in some records the words "stuck together" are used, and in one developed youngster he gives the following percept "2 girls sitting on rocks . . . they look like identical twins." It is important to remember here that for the sample at age 7 being described all of the children are fraternal and this particular boy has two girl siblings, neither of whom look anything alike.

At the following developmental level studied with the Rorschach, we have one cohort tested at age 8, and four of the original cohorts tested at age 9. We have data for an additional cohort of identical triplet girls for comparison at age 9. Cohort 1 (at age 8) had 24 humans, 7 quasi humans, and 2 human details. Cohort 2 had 9 humans, 7 quasi humans, and 1 human detail. Cohort 3 had 11 humans, 3 quasi humans, and 1 human detail. Cohort 4 had 7 humans, 6 quasi humans, and 5 human details. Cohort 5 had 8 humans, 2 quasi humans, and 2 human details. The indentical triplet cohort had 3 humans, 8 quasi humans, and 3 human details. They are more similar to the identical twin girls whom we saw in another context and who at age 7 attained 3 humans, 6 quasi humans, and 6 human details. At age 7, the cohorts reported upon above had 60% humans. At age 9 (except for the cohort tested at age 8) they obtained 62% full figure humans. There may be some stable point beyond which number of humans seen becomes relatively consistent within a particular cohort, with room for development for those with the lowest rate of production.

Of the percepts produced at age 8 and 9, 32 out of 95 or 34% were malevolent, as compared with 16 out of 67 or 24% at age 7. We are comparing children at early latency here with those in middle toward late latency when superego controls are diminishing against expression of malevolent and aggressive fantasy. In reviewing the nature of the objects depicted in this group of records, I am struck more by their similarity from cohort to cohort rather than their dissimilarity. People are sitting, looking, bending, pulling . . . something. There is an occasional more active expression of the activity conflict of this age: "two people firing at each other", "two people shooting", or an imaginative, "two witches casting a spell". And there are benevolent expressions, smiling and laughing faces, people kissing.

CLINICAL VIGNETTES

We will now describe the final outcome of the children we reported upon in Chapter 6. This will be a personality description of the two low birth weight, two middle birth weight, and two heavier birth weight children reported upon in that chapter. We also have followup measurements on the two low birth weight children, and we will report on them at age 12, as well.

Low Birth Weight Children

Girl A.

A. had well developed above average verbal abilities at age 5, and was described at that time as a youngster moving well along in progressive internalization, identification, and control on an appropriate basis. Mother reported her to be the most independent of the cohort. She was thought to give this impression because of her tendency to distance from affective involvement, with the use of control over emotional expression. There was some competition with female siblings and a close association with one of the male siblings at this time.

At age 7, A. continued to obtain above average verbal abilities, with verbal better than performance scores. Her best verbal abilities were in vocabulary and abstract reasoning. In the performance area, her strengths included fine motor coordination and awareness of environmental detail. There were two rotations on block designs, but the examiner felt that if there was a perceptual problem she was coping well with it. She drew a man first in the human figure drawing test, suggesting some identification with more "tomboy" characteristics at this time. On the ink blot test, her percepts were generally happy and socially oriented: "two bunny rabbits about to kiss." Her affects tended to be well controlled, but she was described as tending to act rather than to use fantasy for emotional expression. Her emotional functioning was described as "well-balanced, controlled, and integrated."

At age eight, A. seemed less sure of herself during the testing, but her overall performance on cognitive tests improved in the nonverbal area. The suggestion of perceptual difficulty had disappeared and it had now become a relative strength for her. Her overall performance continued to be in the above average level of intelligence. The nonverbal improvement was also seen in her improved scores on the human figure drawings. Nervousness showed up on an Arithmetic test which seemed to be related to a need to succeed, but generally her cognitive functioning was more even at this age. On the ink blot test, there seemed to be a move toward the use of fantasy, with the development of a rich inner life, but with good capacity to differentiate fantasy from reality. Her ego development was described as appropriate and somewhat advanced. Gender identification was appropriately developed.

On followup testing at age 12, A. was described as "mature, upfront, pleasant and cooperative." She was determined to do well, and she was serious about it. Intellectually, there was a numerical drop in her test scores, which are well within the average range. There was a nice balance in her scores between the verbal and performance scales. It was felt that the numerical drop was related to her approaching adolescence. The personality profile was that of a person "psychologically well intact," with good reality testing, object constancy, and relatedness. She was described as being preoccupied, age appropriately so, with issues of individuation and autonomy. "In sum, she is an adolescent who is currently placing a high priority on becoming her own person."

Boy B.

B. showed exceptional verbal abilities at age 5, but a perceptual motor problem was becoming more apparent, on both the cognitive tests and the human figure drawing test. His best scores were on vocabulary, comprehension, and memory for stories, with above average reasoning abilities. He showed some integration difficulty with the ink blot test, with some delay in forming the human percept, and some difficulty with accuracy. These findings were felt to be related to the perceptual integration problem. It tended to make his record look creative. B. tended toward strong masculine percepts, with some conflict over passivity and activity. He also tended at this time to become highly aroused in social-emotional situations, but there was good ability to control himself, and good evidence of capacity for social-emotional relationships. It was recommended that he be given some remedial assistance to aid in compensating for the perceptual problems noted and consistent structure for the high level of emotional arousal.

B. was seen at the clinic for the testing at age 7 to reduce the interference of distractions in the home testing situation. He attained average scores on the WISC-R given at this age, with a higher verbal than performance score. His strength was on the Arithmetic subtest, where he obtained an above average score. He continued to have difficulty with the visuo-motor integration tests, including the human figure drawing test. What is reported at this age is that the most striking thing that had occurred since the last testing was "considerable growth emotionally." He now had two human movement percepts, one of these with considerable originality, "a football player saying 'hike'." There were some emotionally regressed pulls, such as food responses, and a concern with control of impulses. However, he was better organized, and it was recommended that his dependency needs be met and structure in the environment be continued.

At age 8, he was described as friendly, cooperative, and with an excellent capacity for verbal expression, with good vocabulary and reasoning ability. There continued to be a verbal performance discrepancy with evidence of visual motor integration difficulties. Overall functioning continued to be in the average range. There was some improvement in his human figure drawing scores. There was good reality testing on the ink blot test, and good human relatedness and object constancy. Human movement responses had increased from 2 to 3. There was good relatedness, and an absence of explosive or aggressive percepts. There was still some pull for dependency needs to be met. There was also an indication of the creativity noted in earlier test batteries. B. was reported to use his good verbal abilities, vocabulary, and reasoning abilities in excellent functioning at school.

B. was seen in his home at age 12, where he was friendly and cooperative and very well motivated to do well on the test battery. He functioned at the bright normal level of intelligence on verbal tests, with a delay on the nonverbal tests. His highest scores were in general fund of information, abstract verbal reasoning, and social comprehension. His difficulties continued to be with perceptual motor integration, sequencing, and the manipulation of figure-ground relationships.

The examiner reports: "the projective material portrays a youngster who is emotionally resilient as well as psychologically intact. His reality testing, object constancy, and penchant for relatedness are excellent. The record is void of explosive, aggressive, or dependent percepts, suggesting that he is feeling very comfortable and at ease with his psychological development. When he is confronted with stress, he defends himself appropriately by appraising his situation, and selecting self-protective and adaptive resolutions. His own sense of himself is unilaterally positive and confident. In addition to feeling good about himself and where he is in the life-cycle, he is very enthusiastic about his future development. His sense of humour, modesty, imagination, and most of all, his compassion and empathy for others, make him a very likeable youngster."

Middle Birth Weight Children

Girl A.

A. was tested one month short of her fifth birthday. She was the most composed and poised of her cohort during this testing, with the greatest frustration tolerance. She was described as fearful by her parents, and very complex. She was described by them as very feminine and concerned about how she looked. She did household tasks and emulated and identified with mother role tasks. She said once while washing the dishes, "one day I'm going to be a mommy and I'll have one boy and one girl." Indecisiveness was described by mother who also said that this was a trait of hers, that A. seemed to have what she felt were some of her own worst traits. She was described as bugging mother, but fearful and compliant with father. She was having a problem with fear of going to the toilet at this time.

She scored in the above average to superior range of intelligence with advanced verbal and nonverbal reasoning, but her figure drawings scored below this level. She also drew a boy first, because her special favorite quad sibling drew her first. Her ink blot responses at this age were creative and imaginative, dracula and bat man, and it was felt that she channeled her fearfulness in this way. There was some tendency to become overloaded emotionally and to become anxious when overstimulated. She was handling this with blocking, and anger breaking through with increased overload. The mother was counseled at this time with how to help her with her fearfulness that was showing up in the toilet with fear of loss of body products.

At age 7, A. was tested while she was having a joke with one of her siblings hiding outside the window of the room in which she was being tested. A. was described at this time as having some problems in school. She did not score well in school and was needing some help in speech therapy for problems with expression. She was also showing some reading reversals. She is reported to have benefitted from the special tutoring. She is described at this age as a charming child, whom the teacher adored, hard working, and the most pleasant. She was at this age very popular, peers always calling her, with lots of friends. She is, however, also described as being very nervous about missing a class, getting things done, and she tried very hard to please. She was frightened at this age that she would not find mother in a public place, and tended to anticipate problems. Contrastingly, she is described as having a lot of confidence in certain areas. She was in a ballet recital, and performed with her class, and did well with confidence and with style.

A. scored in the average range of intelligence at this time. Her best functioning was on tests of verbal abstract reasoning. Her human figure drawing scores improved at age 7. Her Rorschach ink blot record showed some anxiety, tension, and fearfulness. However, there was also some increase in ability to control these feelings and to adapt. Her responses were more controlled and both her conventional (popular) responses and her accuracy level improved.

At age 9, A. was described as charming and pleasant, and she put forth good effort on the tests. She was functioning again well within the average range of intelligence. Her best scores were on verbal abstract reasoning, vocabulary, and nonverbal social reasoning, as well as on graphic copying of symbols. There was some slight difficulty on finding missing details, and visuo-motor integration. Her human figure drawings, however did not show impairment and scored again in the average range. They are described as "delightful figures of children her own age." There continued to be a tendency to get anxious and to block in response to anxiety. Those responses given on the ink blot test showed good accuracy level for her age. Although the humans she saw were not in action, there were indicators of good emotional relatedness. She was continuing to have special educational help, and responding well to it. It was wondered whether some of the learning difficulties were related to the emotional indicators noted in both the 7 and 9 year old testing.

Boy B.

At age 4-11, B. was shy and almost subdued with the examiner the first day, but sought her out and was very outgoing the second day. He was described by parents as being physically active, and having a lot of trouble with aggression with peers and not knowing how to interact and join in with them. The parents were also finding him provocative, and a negative attention seeking and control struggle seemed to be going on at this time, about which the parents were counseled during our feedback session. B. was functioning in the bright normal range of intelligence, and he seemed to do well on nonverbal reasoning skills. His drawings were immature and scored low for his age. The ink blot record seemed overwhelmingly to be concerned with phobic-aggressive concerns with some associated depression. He seemed to be most concerned about the mother-child relationship. He was handling his resultant anxiety about these concerns with obsessive compulsive mechanisms, seen in his speech repetitions during the clinical testing sessions. In spite of these anxieties, he was developing a good and adequate masculine identity, and was thought to be handling his fears by passive identifications, and/or ingratiation, probably also seen in his positive relationships with adults outside of the home.

B. was quite shy and inhibited during testing, and was slow in performance of nonverbal tasks, but fluent and verbal on the ink blot test. The parents reported a problem in school at this time and he was being tutored and was also being seen by a psychiatric social worker. The parents felt that his learning difficulty contributed to his emotional problems, because he could see his siblings doing well in school when he was having difficulty. He was also bothered that he was the smallest in his class. However, he was excellent in athletics and very well coordinated.

The present cognitive tests placed him in the average range of intelligence. He showed above average skill on verbal abstraction and social reasoning tests and on visuo-motor integration of puzzles. He had difficulty with finding a missing detail of a picture, and was slow in copying symbols. It was felt that the latter difficulties might have been contributing to his problems with reading. His human figure drawings scores improved at this time. There was also a marked improvement in the Rorschach both in the scores and the content. He saw two human figures, one in movement, and he was more accurate in his responses. The many impulsive responses previously seen had disappeared at this age (on previous testing he saw bombs and volcanoes). There were some unusual thinking combinations which tended to occur in a context of phobic content. However, his controls were better, and he was able to recover more quickly from these feelings than during the previous examination. He seemed to be making good use of counseling and tutoring at this time.

B. was pleasant and cooperative during the testing at 9 years. He tended to be slow and to often complete tests beyond the time limit. He was functioning within the average range of intelligence. His best areas of functioning were on Arithmetic and tests of nonverbal abstract reasoning, with vocabulary and nonverbal social reasoning also good. Other scores were lower because of the time limits. His scores on the human figure drawings were good possibly because this is a test without a time limit. His ink blot tests showed fluency and a balance of responses with a normal accuracy level for his age. He showed a good representation of the human form, and relatedness to people. Some of his responses suggested imagination, while others suggested some anxiety about bodily integrity, with some concern around control of impulses. He was reported to be responding well to continued tutoring. The examiner found this child to be appealing because of his obvious effort and cooperation.

High Birth Weight Children

Girl C.

C. was shy, charming, and more laid back than her brothers during this five year old testing. She seemed more lacking in confidence and less needing to achieve, but clearly as able as they were. She achieved at the superior level of intelligence. Her highest successes were on vocabulary and verbal abstract reasoning. Her drawings were average in score and showed more control than at the previous testing. There was more emotional pressure in the ink blot test. Her accuracy level was not as good as on the previous testing, and the one human percept had disappeared. The examiner wondered if she was going through an emotional upheaval with the pressures of this age. She seemed more fearful and with low self esteem. It was wondered that the boys having each other might have been making a difference particularly since psychosexual issues are important during this age level.

C. was pleasant and charming during the seven year old testing. She showed some signs of tension, and was distractible on the Arithmetic subtest. She gave very long and rambling verbal responses. She functioned at the superior level of intelligence. Her strengths were in the verbal and verbal reasoning areas. She had relative weaknesses in the nonverbal reasoning area. Her human figure drawings showed improvement from age 5 and she was functioning at age in a visuomotor drawing test, the Beery Buktenika Visuo-Motor Integration test. The ink blot test showed an improvement in accuracy level and the reappearance of the human figure, one of them in movement. There was rejection of 2 cards, which she could later respond to upon request. There thus seemed to be some developmental growth, but with some continued emotional pressure, expressed in increased intellectual controls and use of a repressive defense. She still seemed to be socially shy. Some of her organizations were unusual, but these also reflected her creativity. One of these responses she called scary, suggesting her fantasy may at times have been frightening for her. She moved ambivalently from a position of needing dependency supplies, wanting babying, to asserting her independence. This might look like oppositionality, but always within a shy and rather carefully distant position.

At age 9, C. was poised and cooperative. There was some decrease in functioning level from superior to bright normal, with the decrements even across all subtests. The human figure drawings scored somewhat higher for the girl drawing. The Bender Visual Motor Gestalt test showed 4 errors, but it was speculated at that time that this might relate to emotional factors of impulsivity rather than any perceputal weakness. There was an increase of creativity in the ink blot test, with none of the rejections noted in the previous testing. There was great responsiveness emotionally, but with some accompanying anxiety and depression. This seemed to relate to aggressive and dependency issues. This emotional lability (freeing up) in latency could account for the seeming intellectual drop in the numerical IQ scores.

Boy A.

A. was seen by a new examiner at five years. He was very cooperative but tended to become restless as the session continued. This never seemed to interfere with his functioning. This was in marked contrast to the previous testings. His controls and frustration tolerance were markedly improved. He functioned in the superior range of intelligence. His strengths were in the areas of vocabulary, verbal memory and abstract reasoning. His human figure drawings did show a delay in score relative to his age, and below what he achieved a year previously. The drawings showed, however, an increase in control and there was also an increase in control on the ink blot test. He had more humans in his record, and one of these was original and creative: "Two men drinking wine next to a waterfall." His accuracy level increased, and the impulsive responses dropped out. This was somewhat at the expense of increased fears, not uncommon at five. There was an increased identification with the father, serving his need for control.

A. remembered the examiner as having tested him as an infant, and was pleased to see the examiner again. However, there was increasing motor restlessness during this test session, and he tended to give up easily on the intelligence tests. He clearly enjoyed the projective tests more and relaxed on them. Intelligence test functioning was at the superior level on the WISC-R, with a higher verbal than nonverbal score. He had begun having difficulty with Arithmetic, Block Design, Object Assembly, and Coding, in perceptual-motor tests and numerical reasoning. His human figure drawings and Beery Buktenika scores were below his age level, all suggesting some minimal perceputal difficulties. On the ink blot test, there was an improvement in accuracy level, and the phobic responses had dropped out. He seemed to be moving emotionally toward increased intellectual controls, and avoidance of affect in the service of ego control. There were two popular human figures (not in movement) suggesting improvement in internal object representations and inner controls. Some of the issues expressed in the content were gender identity issues, need for dependency supplies, and a movement toward the mother when he feels more stressed; and some continued concern over control of aggression. This sequence is demonstrated on the few Thematic Apperception Test story telling cards administered to him.

He wondered if the boy in 8BM was him because he was also wearing a tie, as an anxiety response to the story he tells of someone cutting somebody. He follows this with a story of a mother hugging a little boy, demonstrating his use of the internalized mother to soothe and neutralize his aggressive feelings (that is, use of the object). It was felt at this time that there might be a perceptual motor delay contributing to difficulty in academic subjects, with continued psychotherapy needed to enhance the emotional improvements in ego controls.

A. was social, related, friendly, and cooperative during the 9 year testing. He was curious about the use of the tests and asked many questions. There was a dramatic shift in the pattern of test scores at this age. His full scale score remains within the superior range, but the verbal and performance discrepancy has now shifted so that performance scale scores were better than verbal scores. There was a sharp decrease in the Arithmetic score. The nonverbal scale showed increases in Picture Completion, Block Design, Object Assembly, and Coding. There was also an improvement in score for the human figure drawings. However, five errors on the Bender Visual Motor Gestalt Test indicated some residual visual motor problems. He had less difficulty in giving responses to the ink blot test, but was still able to maintain control of affect and impulses. There was an increase in ability to reflect and growth in identifications with people. He seemed to be attempting to distance himself from affects to maintain control. There were some feelings of inferiority that he covered with some grandiosity. There seemed to be increased settling down and maturation emotionally. He had stopped psychotherapy at his request, and was being maintained on medication for hyperactivity. The examiner raised questions about whether further psychotherapy might be needed at some time to deal with issues of self esteem.

CONCLUSIONS

We have seen a progression from quasi and part humans to humans in the development of the object as depicted in the Rorschach records. The records demonstrate also the separation individuation phase of development in the progression from malevolent to benign objects, and from phobic aggressive preoccupations to the use of the object to soothe. The records have also demonstrated the active-passive conflict as they have negotiated the separation-individuation phases of development. The stress of these attempts was sometimes expressed in symbiotic references, such as "stuck together" and the description of "identical twins", but these references did drop out and were not included in all records.

At age 5, the cohorts showed variability both between cohort members, variability between boys and girls, and overlap in the types of object representations between cohorts. There was also a trend for cohorts to be productive of object representations or underproductive. The variability between cohorts continued at age 7. By age 9, I was struck more by the similarity from cohort to cohort. With the movement towards late latency, there seemed to be more of a freeing up of superego conflict, and greater expression of both active and benign percepts from all cohorts.

The clinical vignettes were included on the same children described from infancy to three years to demonstrate their further development. They included two low birthweight, two middle birthweight, and two high birthweight children. These vignettes demonstrate the generally good outcome of even very low birthweight children. They also demonstrate that perceptual motor and emotional difficulties were not confined to the low birthweight children. Those with these latter problems were given additional help during the course of the project, and appeared to be adapting well.

REFERENCE NOTES

Blatt, S. J. (1976). Clinical Application of the Assessment of the Concept of the Object on the Rorschach. Unpublished Manual.

REFERENCES

Ainslie, R. C. (1985)*The Psychology of Twinship*. Lincoln and London: The University of Nebraska Press.

Ames, L. B., Metraux, R. W., Rodell, J. L., & Walker, R. N. (1974). *Child Rorschach Responses*. New York: Brunner/Mazel.

Bank, S. P., & Kahn, M. D. (1982) *The Sibling Bond*. New York: Basic Books.

Basit, A. (1972) A Rorschach Study of Personality Development in Identical and Fraternal Twins. *Journal of Personality Assessment*, 36, 23–27.

Blatt, S. J., Brennels, C. B., Schimek, J. G., & Glick, M. (1976) Normal Development and Psychopathological Impairment of the Concept of the Object on the Rorschach. *Journal of Abnormal Psychology*, 85, 364–373.

Exner, J. E., & Weiner, I. B. (1983) The Rorschach: A Comprehensive System. *Volume 3: Assessment of Children and Adolescents*. New York: John Wiley & Sons, 54–65.

Goshen-Gottstein, E. R. (1980) The Mothering of Twins, Triplets and Quadruplets. *Psychiatry*, 43, 189–204.

Hamilton, J., Blewett, D., & Sydiaha, D. (1971) Ink-Blot Responses of Identical and Fraternal Twins. *The Journal of Genetic Psychology*, 119, 37–41.

Harris, D. B. (1963) *Children's Drawings as Measures of Intellectual Maturity*. New York: Harcourt, Brace & World, Inc.

Krall, V., Feinstein, S., & Kennedy, D. (1980) Birth weight and measures of development, object constancy, and attachment in multiple birth infants: A brief report. *International Journal of Behavioral Development*, 3, 501–505.

Pruitt, W. A., & Spilka, B. (1964) Rorschach Empathy-Object Relationship Scale. *Journal of Projective Techniques and Personality Assessment*, 28, 331–336.

Rabin, A. I., & Beit-Hallahmi, B. (1982). *Twenty Years Later: Kibbutz Children Grown Up*. New York: Springer Publishing Company.

Rich, D. G., Greenfield, N. S., Alexander, A. A., & Sternbach, R. A. (1976) Genetic correlates and sex differences in Holtzman Ink Blot Technique Response of Twins. *Personality Assessment*, 40, 122–129.

Terman, L. M., & Merrill, M. A. (1973) *Stanford-Binet Intelligence Scale*. Boston: Houghton Mifflin Company.

Winnicott, D. W. (1975) *Through Paediatrics to Psychoanalysis*. New York: Basic Books, Inc.

CHAPTER 12

Summary and Conclusions

This sample of multiple birth children, some of them born prematurely and with low birth weight, gave us a unique opportunity to study the longitudinal development of such children in the most optimal of environmental circumstances. The fact of the multiple births made it necessary for multiple parenting in the first year of life, affording us an opportunity to observe the effects of this in caring, giving, and nurturing families

The results of the earlier developmental measures indicated that the low birth weight, premature children in our study lagged behind in development during the first two years when scored according to birth age, with apparent "catch up" by 15 months to age two. When adjusted for prematurity, mental and motor scores were in the average range or above. The correction for prematurity, however, has been criticized by some researchers because it may overlook other high risk effects in the later life of such children. We did find a relationship between birthweight and developmental status, but other factors related to this such as intrauterine crowding and lack of prenatal nourishment may contribute to this effect. The increases in score after two years of age may relate to socioeconomic environmental influences and the important influence of caring caretakers and the presence of their multiple siblings.

There was a relatively consistent pattern for mental scores to increase above the level of the motor scale. This did not seem to be entirely a ceiling effect, for some individual children showed increased motor development with age, as scored by the Bayley motor scale. Also, there were children in low and high birthweight cohorts who later continued to demonstrate perceptual motor difficulties.

Our findings indicated that objectal development preceded object constancy in the early infancy of these multiple birth children. It suggested that for our infants in a multiple caretaking situation during the first year of life, that the specific attachment to the mothering figure was not impaired. There seemed to be an adequate amount of mothering available to these infants. The data also suggested that at the early ages, objectal development was related to intellectual development, while later there was a closer correspondence with object constancy as a forerunner of cognitive capacities. Our observations suggested that when object relations achieve some more mature level, both object constancy measures and intellectual development increased, and other factors such as the social environment, SES, and possibly the stimulation of other siblings clearly influenced intellectual development beyond birthweight and other maturational effects.

Our more detailed measurements of the early infant development seemed to suggest that different measures at different ages are predictive of later more complex behaviors. At early ages, simple behaviors of a perceptual motor nature seem to be precursors of later language and cognitive development. At later ages, more adaptive, imitative, and social skills are related. There was a pattern of shift in the measures that related to later language and cognitive developmental level: from motor and perceptual to objectal and imitative functions, and then to vocalization and social-communicative skills. There is growing evidence that the precursors of language are based on earlier experience and abilities to form relationship concepts and to understand categories. There appears to be a high relationship between prehension and motor skills and the development of the object concept and categorical thinking. The gestural imitation stage is also an important precursor to language and highly related to the motor skills that are its precursor. It may well be this movement from action to language and the lesser opportunity for low birth weight children to motorically investigate their environment that has an important influence on the delays in early measures. The delays in motor development noted in the earlier measures may also show its effects in the later development of some of the children.

There has been increased concern that the corrections for prematurity used with early developmental measures are ignoring later high risk effects. There was the "catch up" effect by two years of age noted in our early data, with increases beyond the average level by three years of age. It was suggested that social and caretaker interaction has a greater effect on later outcome as significant as other factors in prediction. However, by school age, there was some reduction in overall intellectual measures in our children, relative to their previous scores. This was at the time of change from the Stanford

Binet, Form L-M intelligence test to the Wechsler Intelligence Scale for Children, Revised at age 7. We questioned whether this could be entirely explained by the change in test.

There were also five targeted learning problem children, all of whom had some subtest scores lower than twice the standard error of measurement for their age group, in comparison with children not so identified, by seven years of age. These findings persisted into the nine year old measurements. The subtest scores most often lower than twice the standard error of measurement were the Picture Completion and the Arithmetic subtests of the WISC-R at age 7, and the Arithmetic subtest at age 9.

While there seems to be some diminishing of the scores between 5 and 7 that persists to age 9, our group tends to demonstrate caregiver and socioeconomic effect. In our sample, the test scores were on the average higher than reported elsewhere in the literature for premature groups and for multiple birth children. The final outcome intelligence measures seemed more equivalent to the high birth weight measures of other investigators. Where there is high risk effect, the greatest deficits reported in the literature seems to be in motor scores. There were some reported learning problems in our sample, and these children showed some difficulties with specific subtests, particularly Picture Completion and Arithmetic on the Wechsler scale. It must be noted that the targeted children having learning problems were not all from low birthweight cohorts. Three of them were from low birthweight cohorts, and two from high birthweight cohorts. These problems were identified early in our regular testing schedules, and many social and emotional amenities provided to enhance their development.

The personality measures reflected this high emphasis on social and emotional development and controls. Affectivity across all ages in our sample showed greater control and less impulsivity as a group than a standardization sample. There seemed to be good movement in the cohorts as a whole toward actualization and neutralization of aggression, and the internalization of internal representations for soothing and provision of both controls and self enhancement. Mentions of symbiotic problems in the personality tests either with primary caretakers or between siblings as interferences with identity formation were few, and disappeared by the latest age studied. Our cohorts were different from each other, and the children within cohorts were also variable from one another, including girls from girls, and boys from boys. There did not seem to be any consistent sex differences.

Many opportunities for differential experience and individuation from parental figures and from each other were given by the families. The follow up data on the one cohort studied at age twelve gives ample evidence of the individuality and adequacy of emotional development.

Such high risk effects that have been seen in the school age data and those children who needed both learning disability help or emotional help through psychotherapy have been distributed throughout the sample, from low birthweight to high birthweight cohorts. It is possible that multiple birth status itself contributes to these effects. That is, that there are subtle factors in the intrauterine environment that affect developmental outcome regardless of the actual birthweight of the infants. And the factor of multiple birth itself as part of the social emotional environment in which one develops contributes to some later difficulties in some of the children involved. However, another viewpoint might be that in any sibship of three to five children, there is room for variability in outcome. We may conclude for our sample as a whole and on the average that these children achieved average to above average status intellectually and their emotional development has proceeded well. We have shown this to adolescence for one low birthweight cohort reported upon here.

INDEX

Note: Page numbers followed by t indicate tables.